ALSO BY DR. STEPHEN PETERS:

Evidence-Based Horsemanship

The Book of Neuropoetry

HORSE BRAIN SCIENCE

THE NEUROSCIENCE OF ETHICAL HORSEMANSHIP

HORSE BRAIN SCIENCE

THE NEUROSCIENCE OF ETHICAL HORSEMANSHIP

DR. STEPHEN PETERS

Wasteland Press
www.wastelandpress.net
Shelbyville, KY USA

Horse Brain Science: The Neuroscience of Ethical Horsemanship
by Dr. Stephen Peters

Copyright © 2025 Dr. Stephen Peters
ALL RIGHTS RESERVED

First Printing – October 2025
Paperback ISBN: 978-1-68111-615-0
Hardback ISBN: 978-1-68111-624-2
eBook available via Kindle and Nook

Additional photographic and graphic image contributions were made by Rebecca Syndergaard, SOMSO Modelle company, and Shutterstock.com

Back cover photo and front cover design by Michelle Snook

NO PART OF THIS BOOK MAY BE REPRODUCED IN ANY FORM, BY PHOTOCOPYING OR BY ANY ELECTRONIC OR MECHANICAL MEANS, INCLUDING INFORMATION STORAGE OR RETRIEVAL SYSTEMS, WITHOUT PERMISSION IN WRITING FROM THE COPYRIGHT OWNER/AUTHOR

Printed in the U.S.A.

0   1   2   3   4   5   6

To all the horses, our teachers who carry us beyond ourselves.

ACKNOWLEDGEMENTS

This book could not have been written without the horses who have carried me—selflessly, patiently, and with their wisdom. They have been my greatest teachers, guiding me beyond and into deeper understanding. I am equally indebted to the people who have stood beside me on this journey, offering their knowledge, encouragement, and belief in the importance of bringing neuroscience to the service of the horse.

A project of this scope is never the work of one individual alone. I am deeply grateful to those whose support, creativity, and generosity helped bring *Horse Brain Science* to life. My heartfelt thanks to Tim Renfrow of Wasteland Press for his support and belief in this book from its earliest stages; and to my wife, Michelle Snook, for her unwavering encouragement and for lending her creativity to the design of the cover and author photograph.

I am indebted to the Sommer family, owners of the 150-year-old SOMSO Modelle company in Coburg, Germany, for granting permission to use photographs of their remarkable anatomical horse brain models. To Rebecca Syndergaard for her stunning brain photography; to Kim Stone for her careful work in labeling; and to Tanja Fichera and Alicia Bajada, whose meticulous proofreading helped refine and polish these pages.

My sincere thanks also go to Dr. Pebbles Turbeville for contributing a thoughtful and inspiring foreword, and to Dr. Andrew McLean for his generous endorsement and support of this work.

And finally, to Kip, my Australian Shepherd, whose companionship on long walks and quiet winter evenings provided both comfort and inspiration—you kept me moving forward.

To each of you, my gratitude runs deep.

TABLE OF CONTENTS

FOREWORD xiii

INTRODUCTION xvii

SECTION I: Foundations of Equine Neuroscience 1

    Introduction to Equine Neuroscience 3

    Anatomy of the Equine Brain 6

    Myelination and Development 47

    Neuroplasticity 52

    Neuroendocrinology 58

    HPA Axis (Hypothalamic-Pituitary-Adrenal Axis) 85

    Long Term Potentiation (LTP) and Memory Formation 88

SECTION II: Sensory Processing, Emotion, and Behavior 93

    Sensory Perception and Processing 95

    Safety First: The Neurobiology of Fear, Stress, and
        Emotional Well-being in Horses 116

    Autonomy and Self Reliance 142

SECTION III: Learning, Training, and Welfare 147

    Learning, Memory, and Training 149

    Environment, Welfare, and the Five Domains Model 156

    Anthropomorphism 186

SECTION IV: Horsemanship Principles 191

    The Principles of an Evidence-Based Approach to
        Horsemanship 193

    Bridging Science and Practice for the Future 200

GLOSSARY OF KEY TERMS 209

BIBLIOGRAPHY 217

A poem by Michael Benner

The Language of Neurons: How Horses Learn to Trust
The doctor stands before the crowd,
His voice steady, like the pulse of a horse at rest,
Speaking of neurons and signals that spark beneath the surface,
Unseen network that shapes fear,
Guides movement,
Teaches survival.
The horse's brain woven with instinct and memory,
Delicate balance of circuits
Flickering between calm and chaos.
Cerebrum holds choices,
Each step,
Each glance,
A calculation of safety,
A flicker of trust,
Or a flick of the ear that signals escape.
Limbic system remembers…
Fear carved deep into synapses,
pattern that repeats itself
Hoofbeats on hard ground,
Eyes wide with ancient knowledge:
Run first, think later.
Amygdala flares,
A match lit in the dark,
And the body follows
Muscles coiled,
Lungs drawing breath for flight.
Yet there is more,
Than flight and fear,

Than the raw surge of survival.
There is the slow building,
Quiet work of dendrites growing,
Reaching out like roots in the soil of understanding.
In the stillness between threats,
The horse learns…
How pressure means release,
How a hand can guide rather than force,
How calm is a path found through repetition,
Through the gentle coaxing of the parasympathetic,
Whispering to rest, to trust,
To allow the world to slow.
Nervous system, a map of balance,
Its currents flowing beneath skin and sinew,
Telling the horse when to move,
When to pause,
When to trust the rider's hand.
The doctor speaks of this,
Of regulation and rhythm,
Of how the horse's heart and brain
Find their way back from the edge of flight,
How each new connection between cells
Becomes a bridge to understanding,
To peace.
And so, we learn too…
Of the power in stillness,
Of the growth in silence,
Of the space we must give
To let the mind unfold,
To dwell
Like the horse,
Each dendrite reaching toward the light of knowing.

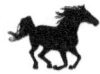

Foreword

My first interaction with Dr. Steve Peters was when he graciously presented a webinar for Horses and Humans Research Foundation (HHRF) in 2024. By then, I had already read the book he co-authored with Martin Black, *Evidence-Based Horsemanship*. If you saw all the sticky notes and margin scribbles in my copy, you'd know just how much it resonated with me. Hearing Dr. Peters present took it to another level. For a neuroscientist who knows so much about the brain, he has an incredible gift: he speaks so clearly that everyone in the room can understand. That's remarkable, because so many researchers and scientists have their own language and struggle to translate research into practical, usable knowledge.

At the end of that webinar, he said, *"Let's remain question driven."* That sentence has stayed with me ever since. Imagine how much more we might understand—about horses, about people, about the world—if we all remained question driven.

Teachers study human development before working with children—so why wouldn't horsemen want to understand the development and "wiring" of the horse's brain before working with them? Observing behavior and practicing conditioning are important but pairing that with an understanding of the brain creates better communication and learning for both horse and human. The science is here, and Dr. Peters interprets it in a way that is accessible, meaningful, and applicable.

This book empowers readers by presenting scientific information in digestible bites that help us understand the horse and improve horse welfare. The more we understand, the more we can increase learning, reduce stress, and become better horsemen. Dr. Peters explains why old habits are hard to break and why consistency is so important in training horses. He gives us both the why and the how in a way that deepens our practice and knowledge.

Understanding the horse's brain, nervous system, and sensory systems (vision, hearing, smell, even vibrissae), along with why sleep is so important, provides invaluable insight into their behavior, learning, and welfare needs. As Dr. Peters explains, tactile perception also plays a crucial role in training and communication between horse and rider. Something as simple as how we pet or groom a horse can either build trust and connection or unintentionally create tension. Knowing how to interact with a horse, especially when we don't know their background or experiences, is essential. Horses are sentient beings with complex systems, and we have a responsibility to understand them in order to truly connect and communicate.

One of the most important lessons in this book is how the horse's nervous system, like our own, shapes behavior and responses. Fear and confusion can trigger the sympathetic nervous system, signaling fight or flight. This is critical for anyone who spends time around horses. By understanding both the horse's nervous system and our own, we can create more efficient training, deeper trust, and ultimately more ethical relationships.

Dr. Peters also incorporates the Five Domains Model of Equine Welfare, offering an evidence-based framework to assess and enhance the well-being of horses. Too often, human needs or convenience overshadow equine needs, sometimes in ways that are harmful, such as isolating horses from necessary social bonds. Knowing what horses require for emotional health and welfare not only makes us better horsemen, it makes us better caretakers of these remarkable animals.

It saddens me that, historically, humans have ignored horses' physiological and emotional needs—at times out of ignorance, at times out of convenience. Horses thrive on consistency and structure, and their welfare depends on our willingness to respect them as the sentient beings they are. As Dr. Peters points out, we are two different animals, but as humans we have the ability to read, study, and apply science to better understand our counterparts. The ethical responsibility rests with us. That means refraining from anthropomorphism: horses are not acting out of spite or meanness. They are simply responding to our communication—or miscommunication.

Even though this book is grounded in science, Dr. Peters weaves through it a sense of poetry that is refreshing and moving. His ability to interpret the neuroscience of horses with both precision and artistry makes this book not just informative but inspiring.

I encourage you to take your time with this book. There is so much valuable content that you won't want to rush through it. You'll take notes, reread passages, and discover new insights each time. The more we understand, the less we rely on forceful or domineering techniques—and that leads to the best possible well-being for the horse. In a time when society is paying close attention to how we interact with animals, *Horse Brain Science: The Neuroscience of Ethical Horsemanship* offers the transparency, science, and ethical framework needed for better interactions whether in sport, therapy, recreation, or simply the quiet moments we share with a horse.

— Dr. Pebbles Turbeville, Ed.D.
CEO, Horses & Humans Research Foundation
2025

Introduction

For over a decade, neuroscientist Dr. Stephen Peters has pioneered the integration of neuroscience into the world of practical horsemanship. His groundbreaking work began with Evidence-Based Horsemanship, co-authored with horseman Martin Black, a book that bridged clinical neuroscience with hands-on horse training. Building on recent scientific breakthroughs, a wealth of empirical research, and extensive practical experience, Peters now presents *Horse Brain Science: The Neuroscience of Ethical Horsemanship*—a deeper, more comprehensive exploration of equine neurobiology and its direct applications to training, behavior, and welfare.

Dr. Peters brings more than 30 years of neuroscience expertise, notably from his tenure as Chief of Neuropsychological Services at a leading neurology practice in Connecticut. His career focused on assessing brain function in patients with diverse neurological conditions, including Parkinson's disease, multiple sclerosis, stroke, dementia, and traumatic brain injuries. Actively involved in rigorous clinical research trials, Peters embraced the principles of evidence-based medicine—prioritizing systematic, reproducible research over subjective opinions. Observing the lack of similar scientific rigor in traditional horse training methods, Peters set out to change that landscape.

As a dedicated horse owner, Peters recognized that many existing studies in equine neuroscience suffered from limited sample sizes, flawed methodologies, or insufficient control groups. This troubling deficit of scientifically sound research contributed to a prevalence of misinformation and pseudoscience in the equine industry, often perpetuated by social media and entrenched biases. Motivated by the critical need for accurate, evidence-based training practices, Peters dedicated himself to translating neuroscience into practical applications that benefit horses and their handlers alike.

Evidence-Based Horsemanship represented a revolutionary shift from traditional, often force-based methods to a deeper understanding of the horse's brain and nervous system. This approach brought a focus on key scientific concepts, such as the role of the basal ganglia in habit formation, the impact of stress on learning and memory, the critical function of neurotransmitters, and the importance of precise timing in training to optimize learning and reduce anxiety. The book resonated profoundly, offering riders, trainers, veterinarians, and students not only new techniques but an entirely new way of thinking—one aligned with the horse's neurological reality.

Now, in *Horse Brain Science: The Neuroscience of Ethical Horsemanship*, Peters expands and enriches this foundation. Incorporating cutting-edge research on equine neuroendocrinology, sensory processing, and brain plasticity, this book deepens our understanding of how management practices affect horses physiologically and emotionally, influencing their learning and behavior moment-to-moment. It empowers readers to apply scientifically validated strategies to build trust, foster learning, and improve horse welfare, replacing force with understanding.

This book goes beyond mere information—it offers transformation. Whether you're a novice rider, experienced trainer, veterinarian, equine science student, or simply passionate about horses, you'll find insights that immediately enhance your interaction with horses. Some chapters will resonate instantly; others will gradually unfold, enriching your understanding throughout a lifetime with horses.

At its core, *Horse Brain Science: The Neuroscience of Ethical Horsemanship* advocates for evolution—in our understanding, our methods, and our relationship with the horse. It invites us to move beyond outdated practices, embracing ethical and effective training rooted in a scientific understanding of equine behavior and cognition. As we become more knowledgeable and thoughtful, we elevate not just our practice, but the welfare of the horse itself.

> "Remain question driven."
> —Dr. Stephen Peters

Horsemanship has long spanned a wide spectrum—from dominance-based methods to approaches more attuned to equine behavior and emotional states. While some traditional practices were forceful, others emerged from careful observation and lived experience, often aligning with principles that neuroscience only now helps to explain. Rather than discarding these earlier insights, modern neuroscience sharpens and deepens them. By understanding the brain systems involved in learning, stress regulation, and social bonding, we can refine horsemanship into a practice that is not only more effective but also more ethical and emotionally intelligent. An evidence-based approach allows us to integrate enduring wisdom with contemporary science in ways that benefit both horse and human.

A Note on Repetition and Language

Throughout this book, certain terms and concepts intentionally recur. Like horses, humans learn effectively through repetition, with each revisit deepening understanding and practical application. Learning precise neuroscientific language can initially feel challenging, but mastering it yields invaluable clarity, allowing for more accurate observation and interpretation of equine behavior. This new vocabulary enhances communication and fosters deeper, more meaningful engagement with the horse's brain and nervous system.

This book bridges theory and practice, blending neuroscience with real-world application. By understanding how horses perceive, learn, and respond, you can adopt techniques that facilitate learning, minimize stress, and build trust. Clear understanding supports your learning journey, sharpening your eye for subtle yet significant behavioral cues.

Every reader will interact with this material uniquely, influenced by their individual experience and knowledge. Regardless of your starting point, this book encourages a scientific mindset—asking insightful questions, honing observational skills, and applying your understanding directly in the saddle.

With this foundation established, let's begin our fascinating journey precisely where true understanding must start, in the brain.

SECTION I

Foundations of Equine Neuroscience

Introduction to Equine Neuroscience

> "Understanding the horse's brain isn't just a scientific endeavor—it's an ethical one. It asks us to slow down, to listen more deeply, and to honor the nervous system—both theirs and ours—as the foundation of every meaningful connection."
> —Dr. Stephen Peters

The Importance of Understanding the Equine Brain

Understanding the equine brain is fundamental to effective communication and training with horses. At the core of equine brain function are neurons—highly specialized cells designed to transmit information through intricate networks. Neurons communicate via action potentials, rapid electrical impulses generated by the precise movement of ions like sodium and potassium across cell membranes. When an action potential travels to the terminal of a neuron, it prompts the release of neurotransmitters, chemical signals such as dopamine, serotonin, norepinephrine, acetylcholine, and oxytocin, into the synaptic cleft—the microscopic space between neurons. These neurotransmitters then interact with receptors on adjacent neurons, either exciting or inhibiting their electrical activity, depending on the specific neurotransmitter-receptor pair involved.

Through this finely tuned chemical and electrical interplay, the horse's brain processes sensory input, coordinates motor responses, forms memories, and regulates vital physiological states such as attention, arousal, motivation, emotional balance, and safety. Despite the complexity and efficacy of neuronal communication within a single organism, direct neuron-to-neuron communication between different species, such as humans and horses, remains biologically unattainable. Consequently, humans and horses must depend upon external methods of interaction—primarily body language, physical touch, vocal signals, and conditioned responses—to establish mutual understanding and effective communication.

Recognizing and respecting these neurobiological distinctions underscores the critical importance of gaining insights into equine neuroanatomy, neurochemistry, and behavior.

The Brain

Everything you and your horse have ever learned or experienced has altered the physical structure of your respective brains. The structure of the brain reflects the environment to which it has been exposed. The experience of the world modulates almost every measurable detail of the brain, from the molecular level to overall brain anatomy. You don't perceive things in the world as they are, you perceive them as your senses have evolved to perceive them. Our brains and our horses' brains are both limited by the specialized biological receptors that perceive signals from the parts of the spectrum accessible to our species.

The functioning of brains reflects how their networks have become organized. Experience sculpts the brain through selective excitation of neurons which shapes functional neural networks. The structure of the brain is constantly changing throughout life. With its billions of neurons and trillions of intricate networks of connections, the horse's brain is amazingly complex. Despite all our current neuroscientific understanding, there is still so much that we do not know and even the knowledge that we think we know remains incomplete. Study of the equine brain is an ever-evolving process and a journey into new frontiers of information and fascination. Every perception, thought, action, reaction, reward, all learning, motor movement happens in the brain. Understanding how the equine brain functions sheds light on why horses react, learn, and interact the way they do. The brain, both in humans and horses, operates as a dynamic, "live wired" system, constantly shaping itself through interactions with the environment. As the brain responds to the demands of new experiences, its circuitry adapts, and its physical structure can even increase in size. Expanding the scope of experiences enriches the brain's capacity for growth and adaptation, a principle that applies universally, including to our equine companions. Every skill that you and your horse have is just a pattern of signals in your neural circuitry.

Anatomy of the Equine Brain

Understanding key directional terms is essential when navigating the equine nervous system. **Rostral** (or **anterior**) refers to structures closer to the face, while **caudal** (or **posterior**) points toward the tail. **Dorsal** indicates the back, much like the position of a shark's dorsal fin, whereas **ventral** refers to the underside. **Medial** describes anything closer to the midline of the body, while **lateral** pertains to structures positioned toward the sides. These terms provide a precise framework for describing anatomical locations and relationships within the nervous system.

Comparative Neuroanatomy

The equine brain, though smaller than the human brain, shares numerous neuroanatomical similarities, reflecting its complexity and advanced functionality among domesticated mammals. On average, a horse's brain weighs approximately 1.85 pounds, compared to the human brain at roughly 3 pounds. Both brains exhibit significant cortical folding, known as gyrification, characterized by numerous folds that create ridges (gyri) and valleys (sulci), with deeper grooves termed fissures. This folding increases cortical surface area—approximately 2 square feet if unfolded—allowing a substantial volume of brain tissue to fit within the skull. High gyrification indexes in both species indicate advanced neurological complexity, particularly when contrasted with mammals like rats, which possess smoother brains.

Central to both human and equine brains is the cerebral cortex, composed predominantly of gray matter—dense clusters of neuronal cell bodies lacking myelination, hence their gray appearance. Mammalian brains universally exhibit a similar neocortical organization, including connectivity patterns from the thalamus and shared neuronal properties. The cortex houses critical motor, sensory, and associative regions, universally partitioned into four primary lobes: frontal, parietal, temporal, and occipital. Some anatomists consider the limbic system as a potential fifth lobe, underscoring its role in emotional processing.

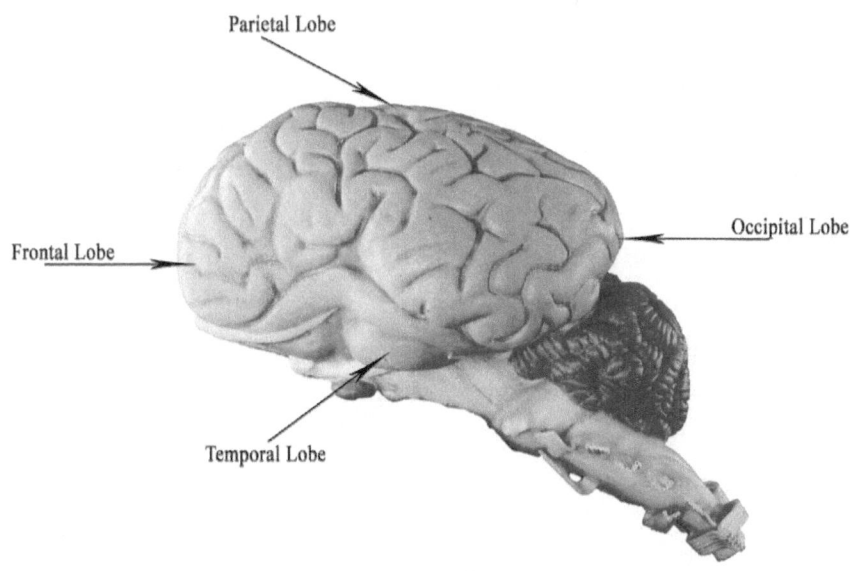

Original SOMSO® model, © Marcus Sommer SOMSO Modelle GmbH, Germany

The **frontal lobe**, positioned anteriorly in the cerebral cortex, significantly differentiates humans from horses. In humans, this region occupies approximately one-third of the neocortex, with a particularly developed prefrontal cortex dedicated to executive functions, including planning, abstract thinking, working memory, decision-making, and emotional regulation. Horses, in contrast, possess comparatively smaller frontal lobes, shaped by evolutionary pressures emphasizing sensory integration and rapid motor responses vital for survival as prey animals. While horses lack the higher-order cognitive capacities such as abstract reasoning or purposeful strategic planning evident in humans, they share essential frontal lobe functions like attention, problem-solving to varying degrees, and voluntary motor control. Importantly, misunderstanding the limitations of equine frontal lobe capabilities can lead to anthropomorphic interpretations, such as attributing deliberate disrespect to equine behaviors. Such misinterpretations can unfortunately justify inappropriate punishment rather than recognizing behaviors as reflections of confusion, fear, or frustration, triggering sympathetic nervous system arousal and instinctual responses like fight or flight.

The **parietal lobes**, located immediately posterior to the frontal lobes, integrate and interpret sensory input. Containing the primary somatosensory cortex, these lobes process tactile information such as touch, pressure, temperature, and pain. They also manage proprioceptive awareness—critical for horses to maintain balance, coordinate movements, and respond accurately to rider cues or environmental stimuli.

Temporal lobes, situated laterally within the brain, house structures vital to memory, emotional processing, and sensory integration, notably the hippocampus and amygdala. The hippocampus enables horses to encode and retrieve memories related to food locations, learned routes, and past experiences. The amygdala is central to emotional assessments, particularly in recognizing threats and triggering adaptive responses. Additionally, temporal lobes process auditory stimuli, crucial for prey animals' survival instincts, and facilitate visual recognition necessary for social bonding and environmental awareness.

The **occipital lobe**, located at the brain's posterior end, functions as the primary visual processing center. Horses possess exceptionally developed occipital lobes adapted to their nearly panoramic vision, essential for detecting predators and monitoring environmental changes. Information from the horse's laterally positioned eyes, highly sensitive to motion and optimized for low-light vision, is rapidly processed here, enabling immediate behavioral responses crucial for survival.

Finally, **the brainstem—including the medulla oblongata and pons**—oversees autonomic, subconscious functions vital for life, such as respiratory regulation and cardiovascular control. In horses, these areas precisely regulate physiological responses, particularly during strenuous activities or stress-induced flight responses. The medulla manages heart rate and breathing, while the pons acts as a relay between the cerebellum and spinal cord, facilitating seamless and subconscious adjustments to environmental demands, ensuring the horse's physiological stability during critical moments.

The Precuneus: Comparing the Equine and Human Brain

One of the most fascinating areas within the medial parietal cortex is the precuneus, a region implicated in self-awareness, spatial cognition, and consciousness. Although present in both humans and horses, significant differences in complexity, connectivity, and function exist between the two species.

In humans, the precuneus exhibits remarkable structural complexity. Highly folded and intricately subdivided, it consists of three major functional regions: an anterior portion related to sensorimotor integration, a central region engaged in cognitive and visuospatial imagery, and a posterior segment involved in self-referential thought processes and conscious recollection. This sophisticated architecture allows dense connections with the **prefrontal cortex**, **posterior cingulate**, **hippocampus**, **thalamus**, and **visual cortices**, making the human precuneus a vital hub within the brain's Default Mode Network (DMN)—active during introspection, memory retrieval, and reflective thinking.

In contrast, the equine precuneus is structurally simpler, with fewer cortical folds and a less differentiated internal organization. Horses rely less on introspective processes and more on immediate environmental awareness and spatial navigation. Consequently, their precuneus primarily supports sensory integration related to body positioning, environmental orientation, and herd dynamics. While horses do possess a Default Mode Network, it is less centrally dependent on the precuneus and instead distributed across other medial brain regions, including the retrosplenial and **posterior cingulate cortices**.

From an evolutionary perspective, these anatomical and functional differences align with species-specific survival strategies. Humans, with an expanded precuneus, are adapted for internal simulation, narrative thinking, and complex social cognition. Horses, meanwhile, possess a precuneus adapted for external awareness, facilitating rapid processing of environmental changes, spatial memory, and integration within a herd—crucial for survival in the wild.

Understanding these differences can profoundly inform evidence-based horsemanship practices. Recognizing that horses experience the world primarily through spatial and sensory integration rather than abstract self-reflection enables trainers to design interactions that align with the equine brain's inherent strengths. Rather than attributing human-like introspection or reasoning to equine behavior, horse handlers and riders benefit from appreciating the horse's specialized neurological capacity for navigating and responding to its immediate environment.

The Integrated System of Key Structures and Functions

Understanding the equine brain requires an appreciation that, while our description will examine individual structures and their specific roles, the brain functions as an extensive, interconnected network. Rather than being a collection of isolated structures performing singular tasks, the horse's brain operates as a complex, integrative system. Each region contributes uniquely to overarching processes such as learning, environmental awareness, and reward-based behaviors. Overlapping functions observed among different regions are not redundant; they reflect the intricate specialization within neural circuits, which collectively enable adaptive and efficient responses.

Though each structure possesses a distinct role, its effectiveness relies fundamentally on its interactions within the broader neural system. For instance, the hippocampus is pivotal in memory formation, yet its function depends significantly on sensory information inputs, emotional modulation from the amygdala, and higher-order regulation from frontal cortical areas. Similarly, reward processing is not confined to dopamine-driven activity within the basal ganglia alone; it also involves cortical regions responsible for decision-making and goal-directed motor actions.

By viewing the brain as an interconnected network rather than discrete, isolated components, we can better understand its remarkable efficiency and adaptability. This chapter will thus explore the specialized roles of individual structures while continually emphasizing a core principle: the equine brain's true capability arises from its connectivity, where each region influences and refines the function of others.

In this section highlighting the key structures and functions of the equine brain, certain essential terms are presented in bold to assist readers encountering these concepts for the first time. This formatting technique serves multiple educational purposes. Primarily, it draws readers' attention directly to fundamental terminology amidst complex scientific explanations. Additionally, bolded terms act as visual markers that aid comprehension and retention, enabling readers to more readily recognize and recall essential concepts throughout the text. Moreover, for readers skimming or revisiting sections, the bolded words offer efficient reference points, allowing quick identification of critical information without needing to revisit entire paragraphs. The strategic use of this visual emphasis is intended to enhance your learning process.

Finally, it's important to recognize that the equine brain, although smaller relative to body size compared to some other mammals, is exquisitely adapted to the horse's specific needs as a prey species. Understanding its integrated nature is key to appreciating how distinct regions collectively shape behaviors essential to survival.

Cerebellum

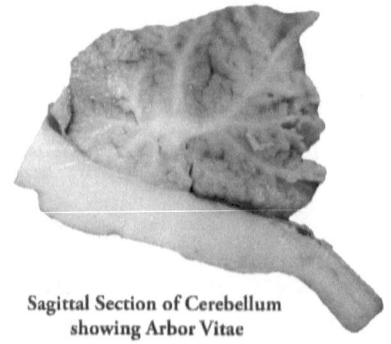

Sagittal Section of Cerebellum showing Arbor Vitae

The **cerebellum**, Latin for "little brain," is a critical structure responsible for balance, coordination, and motor refinement in the horse. It ensures fluid, adaptive movement, allowing the horse to respond quickly to changes in terrain, posture, and environmental stimuli. This structure fine-tunes motor skills acquired through repetition and practice, making it fundamental to the horse's agility, precision, and performance.

The horse's **cerebellum** is located at the back of the brain beneath the **occipital lobes** and is an intricate and compact neural hub. It is densely folded into fine, leaf-like **gyri**, creating a highly ridged appearance that maximizes its surface area. If unfolded, the **cerebellar cortex** would cover approximately three-square feet. This tight folding accommodates an immense number of neurons, more than those found in the horse's entire **cerebral cortex**. This extraordinary neuronal density enables rapid and efficient sensory-motor integration, allowing the **cerebellum** to process and adjust movement with remarkable speed and precision.

In comparison to some other species, the horse's **cerebellum** is disproportionately large, reflecting the animal's need for exceptional motor control. This size is necessary for maintaining balance during fast gaits, sharp turns, and the intricate maneuvers required in various equestrian disciplines. Internally, the **cerebellum** features the "**arbor vitae**" or "tree of life," a striking **white matter** structure that branches through its **gray matter**, facilitating the relay of sensory-motor information to optimize movement execution.

Beyond balance and coordination, the **cerebellum** functions as a predictive processor, constantly comparing intended movements, as planned by the **motor cortex**, with actual movements executed by the body. By receiving real-time sensory feedback, the **cerebellum** detects discrepancies and makes rapid corrections, ensuring precise, smooth motion. This predictive capability is crucial for complex tasks such as adjusting stride length before a jump, stabilizing balance on uneven terrain, and fine-tuning performance in dressage or reining.

The **cerebellum** is essential for **motor learning**. It refines movements over time through repetition, using feedback from past attempts to enhance future performance. This ability to adapt and perfect movement patterns is particularly evident in equestrian disciplines, where horses learn intricate sequences and respond to subtle rider cues with increasing precision. Unlike the **hippocampus**, which governs explicit memory, the **cerebellum** specializes in **procedural memory**, storing learned motor routines that become automatic with practice.

The **flocculonodular lobe**, also known as the **vestibulocerebellum**, is a specialized region of the horse's cerebellum integral to maintaining balance, spatial orientation, and coordinated eye movements.

Comprising the **flocculus** and **nodulus**, this region is deeply interconnected with the vestibular system in the inner ear, facilitating precise sensory integration regarding head position, movement, and spatial orientation. Horses rely significantly on finely tuned motor control and rapid postural adjustments, especially when moving quickly or navigating varied terrain; thus, the **flocculonodular lobe** is vital for their survival. By modulating the **vestibulo-ocular reflex (VOR)**, this cerebellar region stabilizes the horse's gaze during locomotion, ensuring clear vision despite continuous head movement. Neurologically, the flocculonodular lobe processes vestibular input to dynamically adjust muscle tone and posture, maintaining equilibrium and enabling swift responses to shift in balance.

Since horses rely heavily on head position to regulate their center of gravity, any restriction to natural head and neck movement—often caused by overly restrictive training practices or equipment such as tie-downs, martingales, and other limiting headgear—can significantly impair neurological integration. These restrictions interfere with the cerebellum's ability to maintain balance and execute smooth movements, disrupting proprioceptive feedback essential for coordination and spatial awareness. Consequently, this increases stress on the musculoskeletal system and compromises the horse's overall motor coordination.

Riders and trainers should be mindful of how restrictive apparatuses impact equine biomechanics, ensuring that any training aids support rather than hinder the horse's neurological and physical functions.

In foals, early **neurodevelopment** is characterized by jerky, uncoordinated movements that gradually smooth out as the cerebellum matures. The cerebellum undergoes rapid **myelination** soon after initial **myelination** of the **motor and sensory roots**, reflecting its critical role in movement refinement. As the horse gains experience, **synaptic plasticity** within the **cerebellum** allows for the strengthening of **motor pathways**, reinforcing effective movement patterns and filtering out inefficiencies.

The horse's cerebellum is a highly specialized structure that governs movement precision, coordination, and motor learning. Its unique architecture, predictive control mechanisms, and ability to refine motion make it indispensable for athletic performance and everyday mobility.

Thalamus

The **thalamus** is another vital neural hub in the equine brain, positioned deep within each hemisphere atop the brainstem. As a **central relay station**, it orchestrates the processing and distribution of sensory, motor, and emotional (limbic) information, ensuring seamless communication between the body and higher brain regions. This function is akin to an air traffic control center, directing neural signals to their appropriate cortical destinations with remarkable efficiency. Without the thalamus, the brain would struggle to integrate sensory input, regulate motor output, or maintain a coherent perception of the environment, functions crucial to a horse's survival as a prey animal.

The thalamus's fundamental role is as a relay station, processing nearly all incoming sensory data, with a notable exception, olfactory signals, which bypass the thalamus entirely. Instead, olfactory information is processed directly by the **olfactory bulb**, an evolutionarily ancient structure that transmits signals to the paleocortex and limbic system. This **direct olfactory-limbic connection** explains why scent is so intimately tied to memory and emotion in horses. The olfactory cortex, located in the **inferior temporal lobe**, receives input from the olfactory tract and relays it to critical structures such as the hippocampus (for memory consolidation) and the hypothalamus (for stress and hormonal regulation). This specialized pathway allows horses to recognize familiar individuals, whether humans, herd mates, or predators, by scent alone, reinforcing social bonds and aiding in survival-related decision-making.

Beyond sensory processing, the thalamus plays a pivotal role in motor coordination and spatial orientation. The **anterior dorsal region** of the thalamus is particularly significant for relaying head-position information, a function integral to the **vestibular system**. This system enables horses to maintain balance and execute precise movements, whether they are galloping at high speeds, navigating uneven terrain, or responding to sudden environmental changes. The thalamus ensures that spatial and motor signals are properly integrated, allowing for rapid and adaptive locomotion.

A less visible but equally crucial function of the thalamus is its role in regulating wakefulness and arousal. The **ascending reticular activating system (ARAS)**, originating in the brainstem, relies on the thalamus to transmit signals that maintain vigilance and cortical activation. The **intralaminar nuclei** of the thalamus relay these signals using key neurotransmitters such as **acetylcholine, norepinephrine, and serotonin**, helping horses sustain alertness, a critical trait for prey animals in unpredictable environments. The interplay between the ARAS and thalamus ensures that a horse can remain attentive to external stimuli, heightening its ability to detect and react to potential threats.

The thalamus is also deeply interconnected with the basal ganglia, a system involved in initiating and coordinating movement. This connectivity allows for smooth integration of sensory input and motor output, enabling horses to respond to their surroundings with both speed and precision. By working in tandem with structures like the striatum and cerebellum, the thalamus helps refine movement patterns, reinforcing behaviors that enhance agility and responsiveness.

Two key structures within and adjacent to the thalamus—the **lateral geniculate nucleus (LGN)** and the **superior colliculus (SC)**—play an essential role in equine vision and rapid response to visual stimuli. Located within the thalamus, the **LGN** serves as the primary relay center for visual information, transmitting signals from the retina to the visual cortex. However, unlike in primates, where visual processing is heavily cortically driven, horses rely significantly on subcortical visual pathways for survival-driven reflexes.

The **LGN's magnocellular layers** are particularly sensitive to motion and changes in brightness, allowing for the rapid detection of movement, an ability crucial for prey animals. This motion-sensitive processing enables horses to perceive fast-moving threats and react instinctively before engaging in higher-order cortical analysis. While the LGN ensures that visual information reaches the cortex for detailed interpretation, it also feeds directly into subcortical circuits that trigger immediate motor responses.

The **superior colliculus (SC)**, located in the midbrain, works in concert with the LGN to govern **saccadic eye movements and reflexive orientation** toward sudden stimuli. This structure integrates visual input with motor control, coordinating head and neck movements to align a horse's gaze with potential threats. The SC provides a direct, fast-acting visual-motor pathway, bypassing slower cortical processing. This subcortical system enables horses to initiate flight responses instantaneously when startled, reinforcing their capacity for "react first, analyze later" behavior.

This subcortical visual bypass presents an evolutionary advantage but also has implications for horse training and welfare. Because horses are wired to react quickly before engaging in deliberate analysis, understanding their **visual startle response** is crucial for minimizing unnecessary stress. Training techniques that emphasize **habituation and desensitization** help engage cortical learning pathways, tempering reflexive behaviors and encouraging more measured, learned responses. By gradually exposing horses to novel stimuli in controlled environments, handlers can reduce reactive tendencies, fostering greater confidence and trust.

The equine **thalamus is far more than a simple relay station**, it is a critical hub integrating sensory perception, motor coordination, wakefulness, and visual reflexes. Through its intricate connections with the **ARAS, basal ganglia, and visual system**, the thalamus ensures that horses remain alert, responsive, and adaptive to their surroundings.

Hypothalamus

The **hypothalamus**, a small yet profoundly influential structure located beneath the **thalamus**, hence its name, derived from "hypo" (below) the thalamus, acts as the thermostat and barometer for the **autonomic nervous system (ANS)** in horses. This role is critical in maintaining **homeostasis**, the self-regulating processes that stabilize the horse's internal environment while adapting to external changes. By regulating vital functions such as body temperature, heart rate, hunger, thirst, and glucose levels, the **hypothalamus** ensures the horse's physiological, biological, and emotional balance.

When a stressor disrupts homeostasis, the hypothalamus orchestrates a cascade of neural and endocrine responses through the **hypothalamic-pituitary-adrenal (HPA) axis**. It signals the **pituitary gland**, located just beneath it, to prompt the **adrenal glands** to release stress hormones like **cortisol. Cortisol** prepares the horse for the **fight-or-flight response** by increasing **heart rate**, dilating pupils (revealing the characteristic "whale eye"), reducing **salivation**, and redirecting **blood flow** from the **digestive system** to the muscles. This physiological state primes the horse for swift action, ensuring survival in the face of threats. Once the immediate danger subsides, elevated **cortisol** levels activate a **negative feedback loop**, signaling the hypothalamus to reduce cortisol production and engage the **parasympathetic nervous system (PNS)**, which restores balance. Indicators of **PNS** activation include **salivation, pupil** constriction, and relaxed **eye blinking patterns**, signaling a return to rest and recovery.

Beyond stress regulation, the hypothalamus governs several other critical functions, including **circadian rhythms, emotional processing,** and **sensory integration**. For example, it plays a pivotal role in coordinating the **fight-or-flight response** by linking sensory input, such as olfactory signals, to memory and motor functions. This integration allows the horse to respond appropriately to environmental challenges.

The **ANS**, overseen by the hypothalamus, comprises two complementary divisions: the **sympathetic nervous system (SNS)**, responsible for activation and readiness for action, and the **parasympathetic nervous system (PNS)**, which facilitates relaxation and recovery. This dynamic interplay enables the horse to adapt to fluctuating environmental demands while striving to preserve **homeostasis**. Chronic stress, however, can disrupt this balance. Prolonged activation of the **HPA axis** and persistently elevated **cortisol** levels can suppress **immune function**, delay wound healing, and impair **metabolic processes**, highlighting the importance of minimizing stress for equine health.

Hippocampus

The **hippocampus**, named after the Greek word for "seahorse" due to its shape, is a critical brain structure located in the temporal lobes. It plays a pivotal role in memory formation and learning. During the learning process, the hippocampus facilitates the linking of neurons into associative networks by replaying these networks repeatedly.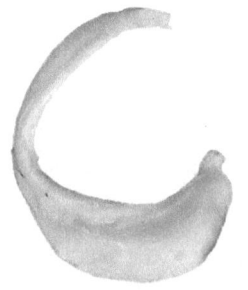
This **replay**, which primarily occurs during sleep, consolidates memories by transferring them from the hippocampus to the **neocortex** for long-

term storage. However, this consolidation process is prone to interruptions, particularly in situations where the hippocampus's ability to synthesize **proteins** is disrupted. **Protein synthesis** is crucial for creating the structural changes necessary to solidify long-term memories.

The hippocampus acts as an **integrator of sensory and contextual information**, bringing together images, patterns, spatial locations, sounds, and other sensory data to form cohesive **episodic memories**. Its plasticity, or ability to create new neural connections, is significantly enhanced by **novelty**. When a horse encounters a novel environment, **dopamine** released from the **substantia nigra**, a midbrain structure associated with reward and motivation, stimulates hippocampal activity. This **dopamine surge** strengthens neural plasticity, allowing the hippocampus to form new connections both during exploration and in the minutes following.

In horses, the hippocampus plays a critical role in spatial navigation and environmental mapping, allowing them to recall the locations of water sources, grazing areas, herd members, and safe routes. Within the hippocampus, **place cells** activate when the horse is in a specific location, forming a neural representation of its surroundings. These cells enable horses to remember the precise location of familiar landmarks, such as a gate, a shelter, or a dangerous obstacle. The **medial entorhinal cortex**, a major input center to the hippocampus, contains **grid cells** that fire in a structured hexagonal pattern, allowing horses to track distances traveled and navigate effectively even in the absence of clear visual cues. Additionally, **boundary cells**, also located in the entorhinal cortex, respond to environmental edges and boundaries such as fences, hedgerows, cliffs, or stream banks. These neurons help horses recognize and remember spatial boundaries, ensuring that they do not stray into dangerous terrain.

As prey animals, horses depend on rapid and accurate environmental assessment, a process in which the **hippocampus** interacts closely with the **amygdala** to regulate **fear conditioning** and

stress responses. When a horse encounters a threatening situation, such as a predator's approach or an unfamiliar and startling object, the hippocampus retrieves past experiences and helps determine whether the situation is truly dangerous.

If stress levels are high, excessive **cortisol** release can impair hippocampal function, making it more difficult for the horse to retrieve memories or learn new information. Prolonged stress can weaken hippocampal connections, potentially leading to difficulties in adapting to novel environments or training scenarios.

These insights highlight the hippocampus' role not only as a **memory processor** but also as a **spatial navigation system** finely attuned to the horse's survival needs. Understanding how the hippocampus encodes and recalls locations, how it integrates sensory information, and how stress influences its function provides deeper insight into how horses learn, how they remember routes and environments, and how emotional experiences shape their memories and behavior over time.

Amygdala

The **amygdala**, named for its almond-like shape, is a crucial structure within the brain's **limbic system**, orchestrating emotional processing, survival instincts, and physiological responses to stress. Located at the anterior tip of the **hippocampus**, it maintains extensive connections with various brain regions, facilitating the evaluation of emotionally significant stimuli and coordinating survival behaviors. While the **hippocampus**, plays a primary role in memory formation, organization, and retrieval, the **amygdala** assigns emotional weight to those memories, particularly those associated with fear and social interactions. This dynamic interplay is especially critical for horses, whose survival has long depended on the rapid recognition and response to potential threats based on past experiences. A horse that has encountered unstable footing leading to a fall or sensed a predator in a specific location retains those emotionally charged experiences, allowing for quick decision-making in the future. Emotional memory formation is vital for a prey species like the horse, as hesitation can mean the difference between survival and predation.

The **amygdala** serves as the brain's central hub for processing and regulating emotions, particularly those of fear, anxiety, and aggression, key components of survival-driven behavior. These emotions trigger physiological and behavioral responses that prepare the body for immediate action. In horses, the **amygdala** detects potential threats through two distinct neural pathways: the **low road** and the **high road**. The **low road** is a rapid, direct route from the **thalamus** to the **amygdala**, enabling an automatic response before the brain fully processes the stimulus. This allows a horse to react instinctively to sudden movements, for example, bolting at the rustle of brush without pausing to analyze whether the disturbance is caused by a predator or merely the wind. This fast, reflexive mechanism is evolutionarily adaptive, ensuring that horses respond to potential dangers without the delay of conscious evaluation. In contrast, the **high road** is a slower, more deliberate pathway in which sensory input first travels to the **sensory cortices** before reaching the **amygdala**. This additional processing allows for a more detailed and context-dependent evaluation of threats. For example, after an initial startle at a flapping tarp, a horse may gradually recognize that the movement poses no actual danger and begin to relax. This dual-pathway system balances immediate reactivity with learned discernment, explaining why some horses spook dramatically at novel stimuli while others, through experience, develop a more measured response to potential threats.

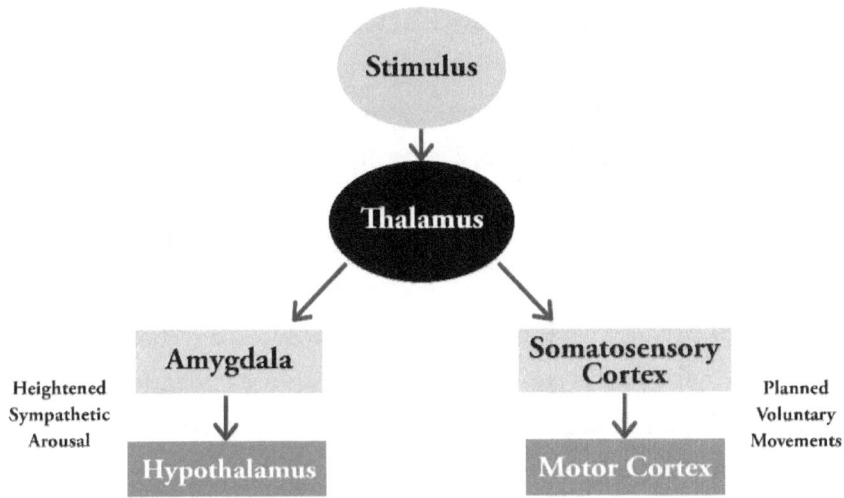

Once the **amygdala** detects a threat, it sets off a cascade of neural and hormonal events to prepare the horse for action. It communicates with the **hypothalamus** to activate the **sympathetic nervous system**, leading to the release of **norepinephrine** and triggering physiological changes such as an increased heart rate, dilated airways, and the mobilization of energy stores, changes that enhance the horse's ability to flee. At the **neuromuscular junction, acetylcholine** is the direct neurotransmitter responsible for stimulating **skeletal muscle contraction**, ensuring that the horse can execute rapid movements efficiently. Beyond its role in mobilizing physiological responses, the **amygdala** works in concert with the **reticular activating system (RAS)** within the **thalamus**, heightening alertness and sharpening sensory perception. This keeps the horse vigilant, allowing it to remain attuned to its surroundings even after a startle response. Additionally, the **amygdala** coordinates with the **basal ganglia** and **cerebellum** to refine motor output, enhancing movement precision during evasive actions. In high-stakes situations, the low road facilitates rapid, instinctual reactions like bolting, whereas the high road allows for more measured responses when the horse has time to assess a stimulus. This integration of rapid reactivity and learned behavior underlies a horse's ability to adapt to changing environments and training scenarios.

One of the amygdala's most essential functions is its role in emotional learning and memory consolidation. Events associated with strong emotions, especially fear, are deeply encoded in memory because of stress hormones, which enhance retention. This mechanism ensures that potentially dangerous situations are not easily forgotten, a crucial factor for survival. However, this process also has profound implications for horse training and behavior modification. When a horse experiences a highly stressful or traumatic event, the amygdala can imprint a lasting fear memory that is resistant to extinction. For instance, a horse that has been trapped in a trailer accident may develop a persistent, seemingly irrational fear of trailers, resisting loading even when there is no present danger. This phenomenon closely resembles **post-traumatic stress disorder (PTSD)** in humans, in which trauma-associated cues trigger intense emotional and physiological reactions long after the initial event. Due to the strength of these fear-based memories, desensitization and counterconditioning techniques must be applied thoughtfully in rehabilitating horses with traumatic experiences. Sudden or forceful exposure to fear-inducing stimuli can reinforce negative associations, whereas controlled, gradual exposure can facilitate the formation of new, positive neural pathways that override prior fear responses.

Although the amygdala is often linked to fear processing, its influence extends to a range of emotional and social behaviors, including bonding, trust, and reward learning. While it plays a critical role in detecting and responding to threats, it is also involved in forming positive emotional associations. The amygdala's connections with the **nucleus accumbens** and **frontal cortex** reinforce social bonds and support learning through reward-based motivation. This is particularly relevant in horses, whose survival in the wild depends not only on threat detection but also on complex social interactions within the herd. The ability to assess and remember past interactions with herd members, trainers, and handlers is integral to equine behavior. A horse that consistently experiences calm, predictable, and positive handling will develop trust and a willingness to engage with humans, a process mediated by the same neurobiological pathways that encode fear. Conversely, negative interactions, such as rough handling or unpredictable punishment, can lead to lasting fear-based responses, affecting the horse's ability to learn and interact positively with humans.

Ultimately, the amygdala serves as a **survival hub**, integrating sensory input, autonomic responses, and emotional memory formation to ensure that a horse can navigate its environment effectively. Understanding the function of the amygdala in horses provides valuable insight into how they process fear, stress, and trauma, offering a scientific basis for training methods that align with their natural neurobiology. Recognizing that the amygdala governs both reflexive fear responses and learned emotional associations underscores the importance of evidence-based, horse-friendly training practices that prioritize trust-building, controlled exposure, and positive experiences.

Limbic System

The **limbic system**, a complex network of interconnected structures deep within the horse's brain, plays a pivotal role in emotional processing, social behavior, learning, and survival-driven responses. Comprised of the **hypothalamus, thalamus, amygdala, hippocampus**, and associated structures, the limbic system is often described as the brain's emotional center. In horses, these structures govern critical functions necessary for adapting to an ever-changing environment, navigating social hierarchies, and responding appropriately to potential threats. As prey animals, horses rely heavily on the limbic system to facilitate rapid decision-making and behavioral responses that maximize their chances of survival.

At the core of the limbic system lies the **amygdala**, a structure essential for processing emotions such as fear, aggression, and social bonding. The equine amygdala is highly developed, allowing for rapid assessment of threats and the initiation of appropriate survival behaviors. This structure plays a critical role in fear conditioning, a process through which horses learn to associate specific stimuli with aversive experiences. Once an association is formed, the amygdala facilitates quick and automatic responses, such as flight or heightened vigilance, ensuring that a horse does not need to re-evaluate a potential danger with each encounter. As negative experiences can lead to lasting fear memories, this function is crucial in training, necessitating thoughtful, positive, consistent training techniques to avoid the reinforcement of maladaptive behaviors. The **hippocampus**, another integral component of the limbic system, is primarily responsible for memory formation and spatial navigation. In horses, this structure aids in learning and recall of locations, environmental cues, and routines. This capability is evident in the way horses can remember precise locations of water sources, feeding areas, and even past experiences with specific handlers. The hippocampus also interacts closely with the amygdala to encode emotional memories, meaning that an emotionally charged experience, whether positive or negative, is more likely to be remembered. This explains why horses may develop deep-seated associations with certain environments, training techniques, or individuals, reinforcing the need for consistency and calmness in handling and training practices.

The **thalamus**, often described as the brain's relay station, plays an essential role in filtering and directing sensory information to appropriate regions of the brain. For the horse, this function is particularly significant given their reliance on acute sensory perception for survival. Visual, auditory, and tactile stimuli are rapidly processed by the thalamus and sent to the appropriate cortical or subcortical structures for interpretation. This rapid relay allows for almost instantaneous reactions to environmental changes, a key feature in the horse's ability to detect and respond to predators. Additionally, the thalamus plays a role in pain perception, influencing how horses experience and react to discomfort or injury.

The **hypothalamus**, a regulatory hub within the limbic system, governs numerous autonomic and endocrine functions, including stress response, thermoregulation, and feeding behavior. One of its most vital roles is its involvement in the **hypothalamic-pituitary-adrenal (HPA) axis**, which orchestrates the horse's physiological response to stress. When a horse perceives a threat, the hypothalamus signals the adrenal glands to release cortisol, a hormone that prepares the body for action. While this stress response is essential for survival, chronic activation due to prolonged stress or poor management can lead to adverse health outcomes, including compromised immune function and behavioral problems. Understanding this mechanism highlights the importance of reducing chronic stressors in equine environments, such as social isolation, inconsistent training methods, and confinement.

The **limbic system's** influence extends beyond immediate survival responses, shaping the foundation of equine learning, memory, and social interactions. Horses, as herd animals, engage in complex social behaviors that require nuanced emotional processing. The limbic system enables horses to form social bonds, recognize individual herd members, and establish hierarchies. It also plays a role in affiliative behaviors, such as mutual grooming, which strengthen social cohesion and reduce stress. Disruptions to these natural social dynamics, such as prolonged isolation or abrupt changes in herd structure, can lead to increased stress and behavioral issues, underscoring the importance of stable and socially enriching environments for equine well-being.

Ascending Reticular Activating System (ARAS)

The **Ascending Reticular Activating System (ARAS)** is fundamental in regulating a horse's arousal, vigilance, and attention, ensuring an appropriate level of alertness for various situations. This system filters incoming sensory information, emphasizing what is most critical for survival and learning. In horses, hyper-vigilance, often linked to stress or anxiety, results in an overactive ARAS, heightening sensitivity to stimuli and increasing reactivity. Conversely, hypo-vigilance, seen in fatigued or overly relaxed horses, diminishes ARAS output, leading to reduced focus and responsiveness. A well-balanced level of arousal is essential for effective learning, excessive sympathetic activation can overwhelm a horse and impair learning, while insufficient activation may cause distraction or disengagement.

The **ARAS** serves as a critical sensory filter, prioritizing significant stimuli in the environment. When a horse detects an unusual sound or movement, this system directs its attention accordingly, enabling swift reactions to potential threats. This ability to distinguish between relevant and irrelevant sensory input is crucial for prey animals, allowing them to survive in unpredictable environments.

Anatomically, the **ARAS** extends through the brainstem, originating from the upper cervical spinal cord and traveling through the medulla, pons, and midbrain to reach the thalamus. The system operates via distinct **neurotransmitter-specific pathways**, each contributing to arousal regulation. **Serotonin**, released from the **raphe nuclei**, modulates mood and wakefulness. **Norepinephrine**, from the **locus coeruleus**, enhances the level of alertness. **Dopamine**, produced in the **substantia nigra** and **ventral tegmental area (VTA)**, is essential for motivation and reward processing. **Acetylcholine**, originating from the **pons**, supports cortical activation and attentional focus, while **glutamate** acts as a primary excitatory signal. These neurotransmitters work in concert to regulate a horse's level of alertness and reactivity to external stimuli.

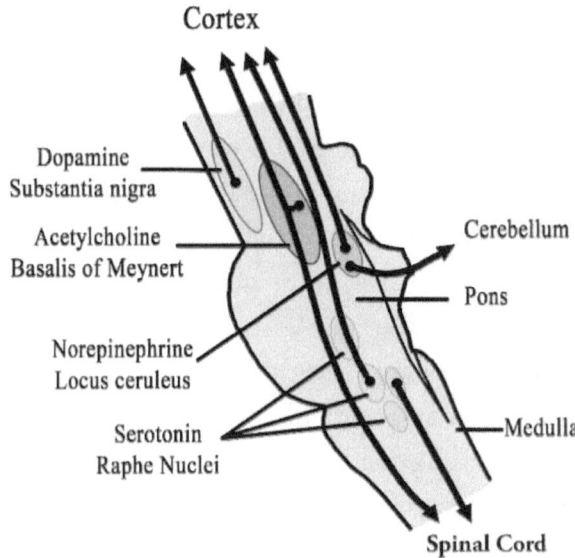

Beyond sensory filtering, the **thalamus** plays a more dynamic role than simply relaying sensory input. It modulates and integrates information from the **brainstem arousal systems** with cortical awareness networks, enabling horses to prioritize sensory stimuli in response to environmental demands. The **ARAS** also communicates with the **hypothalamus**, which governs autonomic functions such as heart rate and stress responses. Additionally, it connects to the **basal forebrain**, specifically the **nucleus basalis of Meynert**, where **acetylcholine** is released to enhance cortical awareness, sustain attention, and support learning.

The **ARAS** plays a pivotal role in a horse's ability to detect changes in its surroundings, such as a rustling bush or an unfamiliar object, an essential survival mechanism for prey species. Its function extends beyond mere reactivity; it also facilitates learning and behavioral adaptation by directing attention to relevant stimuli.

Basal Ganglia

The **basal ganglia** are a group of interconnected **subcortical nuclei** that integrate information from the **cerebral cortex** and influence behavior through multiple parallel circuits. Rather than functioning as a singular anatomical unit, the basal ganglia operate as a dynamic system, transforming cortical input into refined behavioral outputs. This system is essential for motor learning, habit formation, emotional processing, and reward-based learning.

During the early stages of motor learning, the **frontal lobe** is highly engaged, guiding deliberate and conscious movement. As a skill becomes more practiced, the **basal ganglia** take over, allowing the behavior to become automatic, a process known as **hypofrontality**, in which reliance on the frontal cortex decreases as the task is encoded in subcortical structures. In horses, this mechanism enables learned responses, such as gait patterns or reining maneuvers, to become smooth and effortless through repetition and refinement. The basal ganglia continuously monitor sensory inputs comparing incoming information with previously established models, ensuring that motor outputs are efficiently adjusted to accommodate changes in the environment.

The basal ganglia rely on **dopaminergic input**, particularly from the **substantia nigra**, to encode the motivational and reward components of learning. Dopamine strengthens synaptic changes in response to positive outcomes, reinforcing behaviors associated with reward. In horses, this mechanism underlies reward-based training, where reinforcement, such as release of pressure or scratches, triggers dopamine release, promoting habit formation and skill acquisition.

The functional anatomy of the basal ganglia is centered around several key structures. The **striatum**, which includes the **caudate nucleus** and **putamen**, serves as the **primary input center**. The **caudate nucleus** is involved in cognitive processes, including learning, memory, and movement planning, which in horses may relate to navigating complex trails or responding to specific cues. The **putamen**, on the other hand, facilitates **motor control** and **habit learning**, working closely with the **motor cortex** and **supplementary motor areas** to refine movements such as maintaining a consistent gait or transitioning smoothly between paces. The **globus pallidus** and **subthalamic nucleus** act as **key output centers**, relaying information through the **thalamus** back to the motor cortex. This system ensures that motor commands are executed with precision and adaptability, allowing horses to perform complex, coordinated movements under varying conditions.

Basic Circuits of the Basal Ganglia

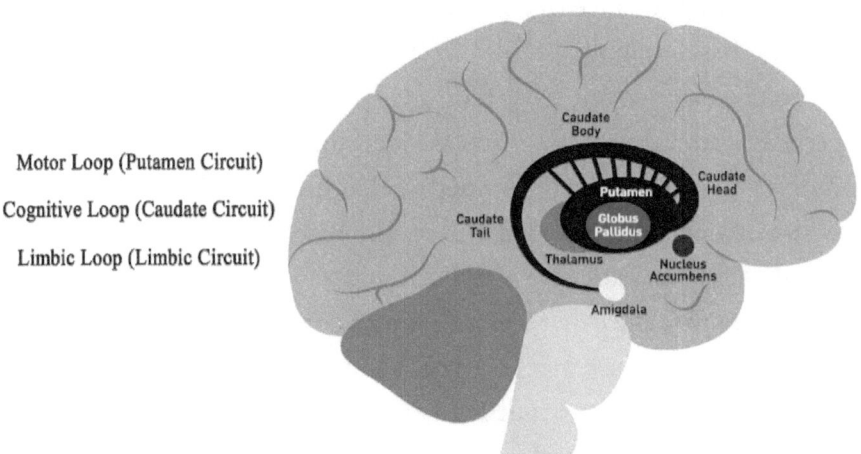

The basal ganglia function through multiple interconnected loops, each responsible for distinct aspects of movement and behavior.

The **motor loop** cycles information from the **putamen** through the **thalamus** and back to the **motor cortex**, refining motor plans to produce smooth and efficient movement.

The **cognitive loop**, which involves the **caudate nucleus**, integrates learning and memory with **action selection**, playing a role in how horses rehearse new behaviors until they become automatic.

The **limbic loop**, connecting emotional centers such as the **hippocampus** and **amygdala** to the basal ganglia, adds an emotional and motivational dimension to learned behaviors, reinforcing actions that are associated with positive experiences.

Horses constantly update their internal models of the world, comparing sensory input with expectations to adapt movement patterns in real time. This process involves **central pattern generators** in the spinal cord and brainstem, which regulate rhythmic movements like walking and trotting. These generators are further modulated by the basal ganglia and cerebellum, ensuring that stride length, balance, and coordination are adjusted dynamically in response to terrain changes. For example, if a horse encounters uneven ground, these systems adapt the movement sequence to maintain stability and efficiency.

The basal ganglia's role in **habit formation** highlights the importance of consistent reinforcement in training. Through repetition and refinement, errors are identified and corrected, allowing motor sequences to be fine-tuned and optimized. Over time, these adjustments become encoded within the basal ganglia, enabling fluid and efficient movements with minimal conscious effort. A horse learning to jump initially relies on **frontal cortex** activity for deliberate planning, but with practice, the **basal ganglia** automate the sequence, allowing for smooth and confident execution.

Ultimately, the **basal ganglia act as a "selection machine,"** enabling efficient, goal-directed behaviors while suppressing competing actions. Through the integration of motor, cognitive, and emotional circuits, they refine voluntary movement, support learning, and facilitate habit formation. In horses, the basal ganglia ensure that practiced behaviors, whether navigating an obstacle course or maintaining a collected canter, become streamlined and effortless.

Ventral Pallidum

The **ventral pallidum**, a critical component of the **basal ganglia**, serves as a central hub in the brain's reward circuitry, integrating reward signals to regulate cognitive, emotional, and motor processes. This structure plays a fundamental role in **motivational salience**, the ability to prioritize and respond to rewarding or significant stimuli in the environment. In essence, the ventral pallidum is responsible for directing attention and energy toward goal-directed behaviors, ensuring that an animal can efficiently seek out and respond to rewarding stimuli while avoiding aversive ones.

In horses, the ventral pallidum is particularly important for processing stimuli related to survival and well-being, such as locating food, engaging in social bonding, or responding appropriately to potential threats.

Corpus Callosum and Anterior Commissure

The **corpus callosum** and **anterior commissure** are critical white matter structures responsible for **interhemispheric communication**, ensuring functional integration between the left and right cerebral hemispheres. The **corpus callosum**, the largest commissural fiber bundle in the mammalian brain, consists of myelinated axons that facilitate the rapid transfer of sensory, motor, and cognitive information between hemispheres. It is topographically organized, with its **genu** primarily connecting frontal regions, the body linking sensorimotor and parietal areas, and the **splenium** integrating visual and posterior cortical processing. However, in horses, the **corpus callosum** is relatively less robust and smaller in proportion to total brain volume than in some other species, such as primates and carnivores. This structural difference may reflect differences in cognitive processing, as equine behavior relies heavily on subcortical and cerebellar structures for motor coordination and decision-making rather than extensive cortical integration.

The **anterior commissure**, while significantly smaller than the **corpus callosum**, serves as an essential bridge for interhemispheric transfer, particularly for **temporal lobe** structures, including the amygdala and olfactory regions. It is one of the oldest commissural pathways in evolutionary terms and is particularly well-developed in species with strong **olfactory reliance**. In horses, where olfaction plays a critical role in social communication, recognition, and environmental awareness, the **anterior commissure** likely facilitates bilateral processing of olfactory cues, ensuring seamless integration of scent-based information between hemispheres. This structure also connects limbic regions, suggesting a role in emotional regulation and associative memory, both of which are highly relevant in equine behavior and training.

Given that the **corpus callosum** is relatively less robust in horses, they may exhibit more **functional lateralization**, relying more on **ipsilateral** (same side of the brain) **cortical and subcortical processing** than on interhemispheric transfer.

The **anterior commissure**, with its **strong limbic and olfactory connections**, likely plays a compensatory role in facilitating interhemispheric communication, particularly in processing social and emotional cues. Given that horses rely on **olfaction and limbic-driven behavior** for recognizing individuals, assessing threats, and navigating social interactions, the **anterior commissure** may play a role in maintaining emotional and social cohesion within the herd.

Overall, the **corpus callosum** and **anterior commissure** form the **neural infrastructure** that supports bilateral sensory, motor, and cognitive processing in horses, though with **species-specific adaptations**. While the **corpus callosum** is relatively smaller than in some species, the **anterior commissure** may compensate by enhancing limbic and olfactory communication.

Internal Capsule

The **internal capsule** is a critical subcortical white matter structure that serves as a bidirectional communication highway between the **cerebral cortex** and other regions of the **central nervous system (CNS)**. Composed of densely packed **myelinated fibers**, it traverses the **basal ganglia**, acting as a conduit for both motor and sensory signals. Anatomically, it divides the **caudate nucleus** and **thalamus** medially from the **putamen** and **globus pallidus** laterally, ensuring efficient integration of motor commands, sensory processing, and associative functions. Functionally, the internal capsule plays a crucial role in linking the **cerebral hemispheres** with the brainstem and spinal cord, facilitating movement, perception, and cognition.

Structurally, the internal capsule is divided into distinct regions based on its shape and fiber organization. The **anterior limb**, located between the **caudate nucleus** and the **lentiform nucleus** (putamen and globus pallidus), primarily mediates communication between the **thalamus** and the **frontal cortex**, playing a role in cognitive processing and decision-making. The **genu**, or bend of the internal capsule, houses **corticobulbar fibers**, which connect the **motor cortex** with **cranial nerve nuclei**, essential for voluntary movements of the face, head, and neck. The **posterior limb**, situated between the **thalamus** and the **lentiform nucleus**, carries **corticospinal fibers (pathways of communication between the cortex and the spinal cord)** crucial for motor control of the limbs and trunk, as well as ascending sensory fibers that relay somatosensory information to the cortex.

In horses, as in other mammals, the internal capsule is fundamental to motor coordination, sensory processing, and learned behaviors. Given their reliance on precise motor control and sensory integration for locomotion, balance, and spatial awareness, the integrity of the **internal capsule** is essential for neurological function. Unlike primates, where fine motor control of the hands is highly specialized, horses depend on **coordinated limb movement**, requiring robust **corticospinal pathways** within the **posterior limb** of the internal capsule. Furthermore, proprioception and vestibular input are critical for equine movement and posture, making the sensory tracts of the internal capsule indispensable for relaying information about body position and environmental interactions.

Cingulate Gyrus

The **cingulate gyrus** in horses has critical connections with the **limbic system**, and is strategically located above the **corpus callosum**, which is the primary fiber tract connecting the brain's hemispheres. This anatomical positioning makes the cingulate gyrus an essential integrative hub, bridging cortical and subcortical regions to regulate emotional, cognitive, and behavioral processes. Specifically, in horses, the cingulate gyrus contributes profoundly to emotional processing, the evaluation of environmental stimuli, and the modulation of responses vital for survival, learning, and social dynamics.

A significant aspect of the cingulate gyrus's function involves the **anterior cingulate cortex (ACC)**, which, alongside the **insula**, forms a crucial part of the **brain's saliency network**. This network is responsible for detecting and prioritizing stimuli that are relevant or significant, thus guiding attention, behavior, and physiological responses. Due to this highly sensitive saliency system, even subtle inconsistencies or mixed signals in horsemanship can feel notably jarring or stressful to horses, who are finely attuned to detecting incongruities as a survival mechanism. The **ACC's** connections with regions such as the **amygdala** and **hypothalamus** further reinforce its role in emotional regulation, error detection, conflict monitoring, and reward anticipation. These functions are critical for a horse's adaptability during training, stress management, and cooperation in social contexts, allowing the animal to adjust its behavior based on the outcomes of previous experiences.

Complementing the **ACC**, the **posterior cingulate cortex (PCC)** plays a pivotal role in spatial awareness, sensory integration, and contextual processing of environmental stimuli. Given horses' status as prey animals, their survival hinges on acute situational awareness and rapid threat assessment—functions supported by the PCC. The ability of horses to quickly recognize familiar settings, anticipate dangers, and adapt their movements accordingly is largely facilitated by the PCC. Furthermore, the PCC's involvement in self-referential processing indicates that horses possess an internal capacity to track experiences and recall past events, leveraging this memory to inform current behaviors and decisions.

Anatomically, the cingulate gyrus's extensive connectivity with critical brain structures such as the **amygdala, nucleus accumbens, hippocampus**, and spinal cord underscores its central role in emotion regulation, attention allocation, and performance monitoring. Longitudinal connections between anterior and posterior regions enable seamless integration of past experiences with present decision-making, promoting behavioral flexibility and adaptability. This sophisticated neural architecture underpins horses' ability to learn efficiently, navigate social hierarchies, and respond effectively to training methods that are consistent, clear, and aligned with their neurobiological sensitivities.

In summary, the cingulate gyrus, particularly through the functioning of the **ACC** and **PCC** within the **saliency network**, profoundly influences emotional, cognitive, and behavioral responses in horses. Recognizing its sensitivity helps explain why horses react intensely to inconsistencies in training, emphasizing the importance of precise, predictable interactions.

Periaqueductal Gray Area

The **periaqueductal gray (PAG)**, (from the Latin *peri-* meaning "around"), is located in the brain stem and surrounds the **cerebral aqueduct** (a cerebral spinal fluid filled duct running through the midbrain). It is a key structure involved in pain perception and modulation, often referred to as an "analgesic center." The **PAG** plays a critical role in a horse's response to threatening, stressful, or painful stimuli, including the initiation of defensive behaviors.

The **PAG** is integral to pain modulation. It receives **nociceptive (pain) signals** and activates the **endogenous opioid system**, which suppresses pain and helps manage its perception during stressful or threatening situations. In addition to modulating pain, the **PAG** is heavily involved in coordinating defensive responses to threats. For example, pain or perceived danger can trigger aggression as a defensive mechanism. These defensive reactions include sympathetic responses such as increased **heart rate (tachycardia)**, elevated **blood pressure (hypertension)**, and rapid, shallow breathing. Such reactions are mediated by the **caudal columns** of the **PAG**. In contrast, activation of the **ventrolateral portion** of the **PAG** through signals from the amygdala produces behavioral arrest, or "freezing," characterized by **hypo-reactivity**, reduced **heart rate (bradycardia), low blood pressure (hypotension)**, and **analgesia**.

The neurochemical activity within the **PAG** also contributes to its role in pain and stress responses. Sections within the **PAG** contain high concentrations of **norepinephrine**, which heighten arousal and vigilance in response to pain. Painful stimuli can deplete **dopamine** levels and reduce the sensitivity of dopamine neurons. This depletion has significant behavioral implications, as a horse experiencing pain may find it difficult to perceive rewards, making training and learning more challenging.

The **PAG's** involvement in regulating defensive behaviors and pain responses highlights the importance of addressing physical discomfort when working with horses. Behavioral signs such as **quiescence**, **hyporeactivity**, or aggression may reflect **PAG activation** due to pain or stress. When a horse is in pain, its neurobiological systems prioritize survival and defense over other activities, such as engaging in training or seeking rewards.

Ventricles and Cerebrospinal Fluid

The **ventricular system** of the brain comprises a network of interconnected, fluid-filled cavities that play a crucial role in cerebrospinal fluid (**CSF**) production, circulation, and homeostasis. These structures include the **lateral ventricles**, **third ventricle**, **fourth ventricle**, and **cerebral aqueduct**. The **lateral ventricles**, C-shaped cavities located in each cerebral hemisphere, are the largest of the ventricles and serve as the primary site for CSF production, facilitated by the **choroid plexus**. CSF flows from the lateral ventricles into the **third ventricle**, a midline structure situated between the right and left thalamic regions. From there, it passes through the **cerebral aqueduct**, a narrow channel traversing the midbrain, ensuring continuous CSF movement. The **fourth ventricle**, positioned between the pons and cerebellum, serves as a gateway for CSF to flow into the spinal canal and **subarachnoid space**, enveloping the brain and spinal cord.

CSF, a clear, nutrient-rich fluid, is vital for brain function, acting as both a transport medium for nutrients and a waste clearance system that removes metabolic byproducts and toxins. Additionally, it provides mechanical protection, suspending the brain in a shock-absorbing fluid that helps minimize injury from movement or impact. This is particularly significant in species like horses, where rapid acceleration, deceleration, and head movements, whether during locomotion or sudden shifts in balance exert considerable forces on the brain.

In horses, the **ventricular system** mirrors that of humans in function but is adapted to the equine brain's unique proportions and structure.

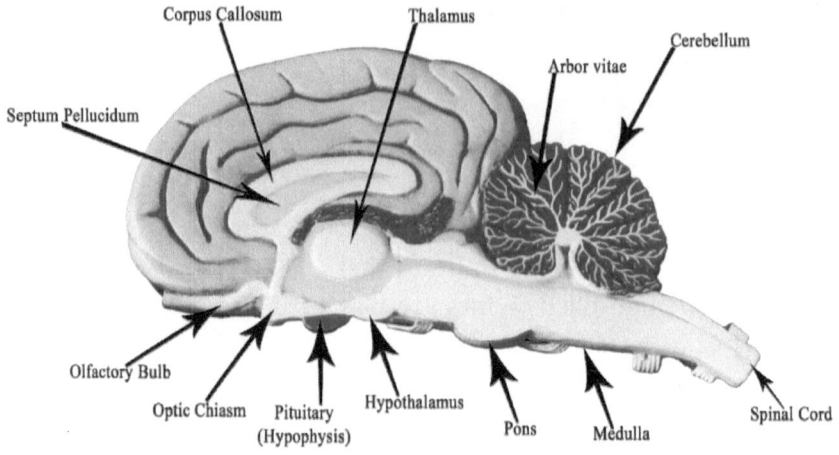

Original SOMSO® model, © Marcus Sommer SOMSO Modelle GmbH, Germany

Cranial Nerves

The horse's cranial nerves are a collection of twelve paired nerves that emerge from the brain, midbrain, and brainstem, playing a crucial role in sensory and motor functions. These nerves primarily serve the head and neck, though some extend to internal organs, facilitating essential physiological processes. Each cranial nerve is designated by a Roman numeral and classified as sensory (involved in perception), motor (controlling movement), or mixed (both sensory and motor). Horses and humans have the same cranial nerves, reflecting the fundamental similarities in mammalian neuroanatomy.

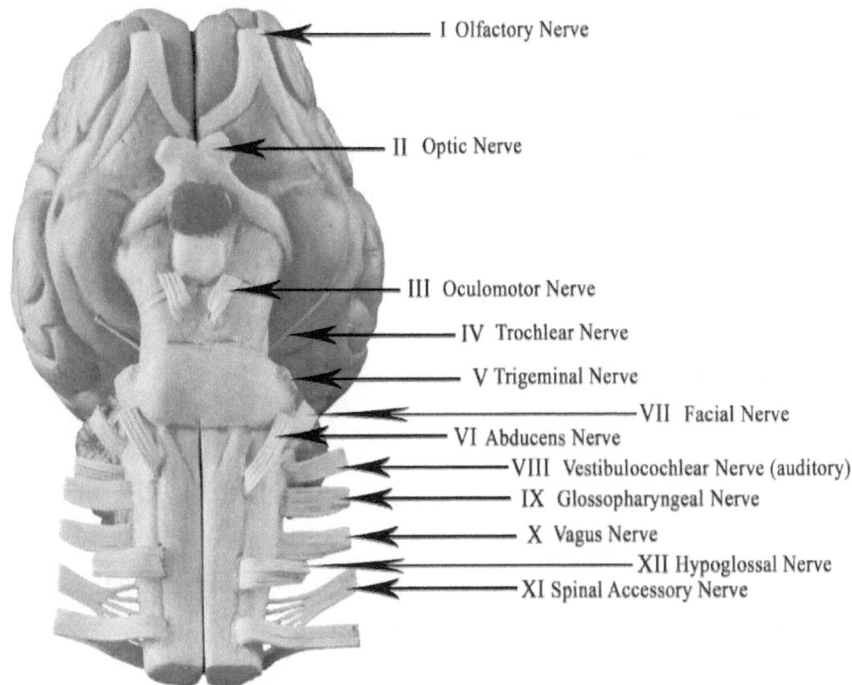

Original SOMSO® model, © Marcus Sommer SOMSO Modelle GmbH, Germany

Sensory Cranial Nerves

Olfactory Nerve (Cranial Nerve I) – A purely sensory nerve responsible for the sense of smell. It detects chemical signals in the nasal mucosa and transmits them to the olfactory bulb. This function is vital for the horse's ability to detect scents in its environment, including food and potential threats.

Optic Nerve (Cranial Nerve II) – Another sensory nerve, the optic nerve transmits visual information from the retina to the brain. Vision is critical for horses as prey animals, providing them with a wide field of view and the ability to detect motion from great distances.

Vestibulocochlear Nerve (Cranial Nerve VIII) – This sensory nerve has two components: the vestibular branch, which maintains balance and spatial orientation, and the cochlear branch, which transmits auditory information from the inner ear to the brain. Proper function of this nerve is essential for a horse's coordination and ability to respond to sound cues.

Motor Cranial Nerves

Oculomotor Nerve (Cranial Nerve III) – A motor nerve responsible for controlling most of the eye's movements, including the superior, inferior, and medial rectus muscles, as well as the inferior oblique muscle. It also regulates pupil constriction through parasympathetic fibers, helping the horse adjust to changing light conditions.

Trochlear Nerve (Cranial Nerve IV) – This motor nerve innervates the superior oblique muscle, allowing the eye to rotate downward and laterally. This movement contributes to a horse's ability to maintain focus while moving.

Abducens Nerve (Cranial Nerve VI) – A motor nerve that controls the lateral rectus muscle, enabling lateral movement of the eye. This function is crucial for tracking objects in a horse's peripheral vision.

Accessory Nerve (Cranial Nerve XI) – This motor nerve innervates muscles involved in neck and shoulder movement, including the trapezius and sternocephalicus muscles. These movements are essential for head positioning and overall locomotion.

FOUNDATIONS OF EQUINE NEUROSCIENCE

Hypoglossal Nerve (Cranial Nerve XII) – A motor nerve responsible for controlling the intrinsic and extrinsic muscles of the tongue, facilitating feeding, drinking, and swallowing.

Mixed (Sensory and Motor) Cranial Nerves

Trigeminal Nerve (Cranial Nerve V) – A large mixed nerve with three divisions: the ophthalmic, maxillary, and mandibular branches. The sensory components provide sensation to the face, nasal cavity, and mouth, while the motor components control the muscles of mastication, enabling chewing.

'Facial Nerve (Cranial Nerve VII) – This mixed nerve governs facial expressions by innervating facial muscles. Its sensory component provides taste sensation from the anterior two-thirds of the tongue, while its autonomic fibers regulate lacrimal (tear) and salivary gland function.

Glossopharyngeal Nerve (Cranial Nerve IX) – A mixed nerve involved in multiple functions. Sensory fibers provide sensation to the pharynx, tongue, and carotid body, while motor fibers control part of the pharyngeal musculature. Autonomic parasympathetic fibers activate the salivary gland, resulting in "licking and chewing," which are commonly observed behaviors in relaxed or learning states.

Vagus Nerve (Cranial Nerve X) – A critical mixed nerve that extends beyond the head and neck to innervate the heart, lungs, and digestive tract. Sensory fibers provide sensation to the ear, throat, and visceral organs, while motor fibers regulate muscles of the larynx and pharynx, facilitating swallowing and vocalization. The vagus nerve plays a major role in parasympathetic regulation, controlling heart rate, respiration, and digestion.

Summary of Cranial Nerve Functions

Motor Nerves: Oculomotor (III), Trochlear (IV), Abducens (VI), Accessory (XI), Hypoglossal (XII).
Sensory Nerves: Olfactory (I), Optic (II), Vestibulocochlear (VIII).
Mixed Nerves: Trigeminal (V), Facial (VII), Glossopharyngeal (IX), Vagus (X).

A commonly used mnemonic for recalling the twelve cranial nerves in order: "On Old Olympus' Towering Top, A Famous Viking Gallops Valiantly Across Hills." In this phrase, each initial letter corresponds sequentially to the twelve cranial nerves.

1. Olfactory (I) – Smell
2. Optic (II) – Vision
3. Oculomotor (III) – Eye movement and pupil constriction
4. Trochlear (IV) – Eye movement (superior oblique muscle)
5. Trigeminal (V) – Facial sensation and mastication
6. Abducens (VI) – Lateral eye movement
7. Facial (VII) – Facial expressions, taste (anterior 2/3 of tongue)
8. Vestibulocochlear (VIII) – Balance and hearing
9. Glossopharyngeal (IX) – Taste (posterior 1/3 of tongue), swallowing
10. Vagus (X) – Autonomic control of heart, lungs, digestion, voice
11. Spinal Accessory (XI) – Neck and shoulder movement
12. Hypoglossal (XII) – Tongue movement

Hyoid Apparatus

The **hyoid apparatus** in horses, though not a neuroanatomical structure itself, occupies a pivotal anatomical and functional position, profoundly influencing equine biomechanics, sensory processing, and neurological integration. Comprising a series of small, interconnected bones—including the **stylohyoid, ceratohyoid, basihyoid, thyrohyoid**, and **epihyoid** bones—the hyoid apparatus serves as a central anchor suspended within the head and neck, positioned strategically between the mandible, tongue, pharynx, larynx, and the base of the skull via connections to the temporal bone. Functionally, it supports essential movements such as swallowing, breathing, vocalization, and mastication, and plays a significant role in balance, posture, and proprioception. Due to its numerous muscular attachments—including connections to the tongue, sternum, and shoulder girdle (via the **omohyoid** muscle)—the hyoid exerts substantial influence on head carriage, cervical alignment, and the broader muscular and fascial chains extending throughout the horse's body.

Disruptions or tensions within the hyoid apparatus can propagate along fascial planes, impacting movement fluidity, postural stability, and proprioceptive accuracy. From a neuroscience perspective, the integrity and freedom of movement within the hyoid directly impact sensory feedback mechanisms involving proprioceptive and vestibular pathways. It closely interacts with cranial nerves—including the **hypoglossal nerve (XII)**, which innervates tongue musculature, and branches of the **glossopharyngeal (IX)** and **vagus (X)** nerves, critical in swallowing, respiratory control, and autonomic balance. Dysfunction or restriction within the hyoid can lead to altered proprioceptive inputs, compromised respiratory and swallowing efficiency, and disturbed equilibrium due to interference in vestibular signaling pathways. Such alterations can result in compensatory muscular tension, increased sympathetic nervous system arousal, stress responses, behavioral disturbances, and impaired learning capabilities.

Importantly, the delicate and relatively fragile nature of the hyoid apparatus makes it vulnerable to injury from rough or forceful handling. Excessive pulling, abrupt movements, strong rein pressure, restrictive tack, or harsh training techniques can easily strain, fracture, or damage these small, interconnected bones and their associated soft tissues. Damage to the hyoid apparatus can cause significant pain, chronic inflammation, impaired biomechanical function, and long-lasting disruptions in neurological signaling, severely compromising the horse's overall welfare, performance, and behavioral balance. Understanding the fragility and significance of the hyoid apparatus underscores the importance of employing gentle, evidence-based training practices that respect equine anatomical and neurological integrity.

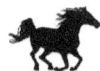

Myelination and Development

Myelination and Neurodevelopment in Horses

Horses are born remarkably well-prepared for life, a stark contrast to human infants, who require years of brain development to achieve even basic locomotion. This advanced state of readiness is an evolutionary necessity, within hours of birth, a foal must stand, walk, and remain close to its mother and the herd for protection. This rapid neuromuscular coordination is made possible by the process of **myelination**, a critical aspect of neurodevelopment that ensures the efficient transmission of signals across neural pathways.

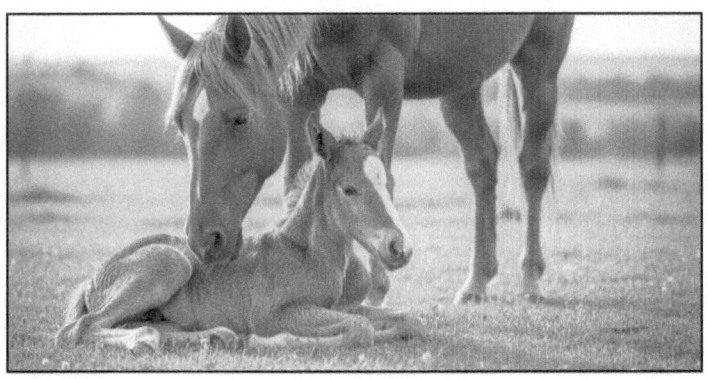

Myelination is facilitated by **oligodendrocytes**, specialized glial cells that wrap nerve fibers in myelin, a fatty insulating substance. This process is akin to paving a highway: well-myelinated pathways allow neural signals to travel swiftly and efficiently, reducing transmission delays and increasing precision in movement. The heavily myelinated regions of the brain, collectively referred to as **white matter**, appear light-colored due to the high fat content of myelin. In foals, myelination progresses rapidly in the first 40–50 days of life, prioritizing the motor and sensory pathways essential for immediate survival. The rapid wiring of these pathways ensures that a foal can coordinate movement, balance, and reflexive responses shortly after birth.

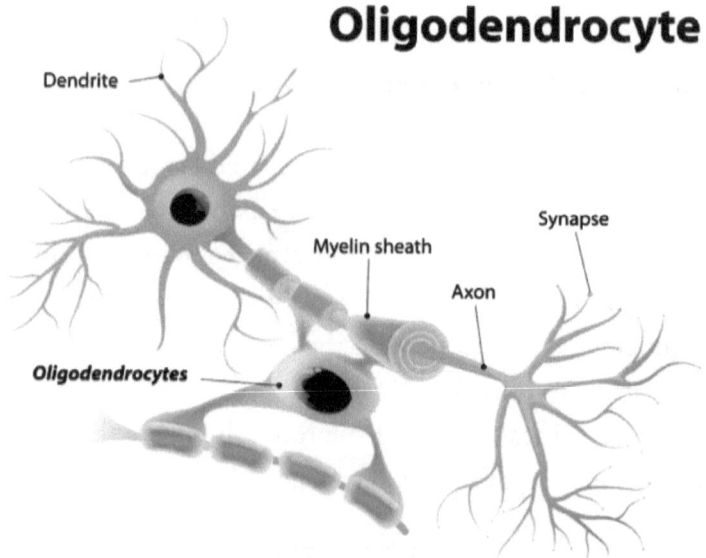

Movement as a Driver of Myelination

Neurodevelopment in horses is not solely dictated by genetic programming, environmental stimuli, particularly movement, plays an integral role. From the very first day of life, foals engage in frequent stretching and exploratory movements, with research estimating that they perform nearly 100 stretches per day by the third day of life. These early movements stimulate motor pathways, activating glutamate-releasing neurons that, in turn, attract oligodendrocytes to initiate myelination. Repeated motor patterns reinforce these connections, accelerating the maturation of motor circuits.

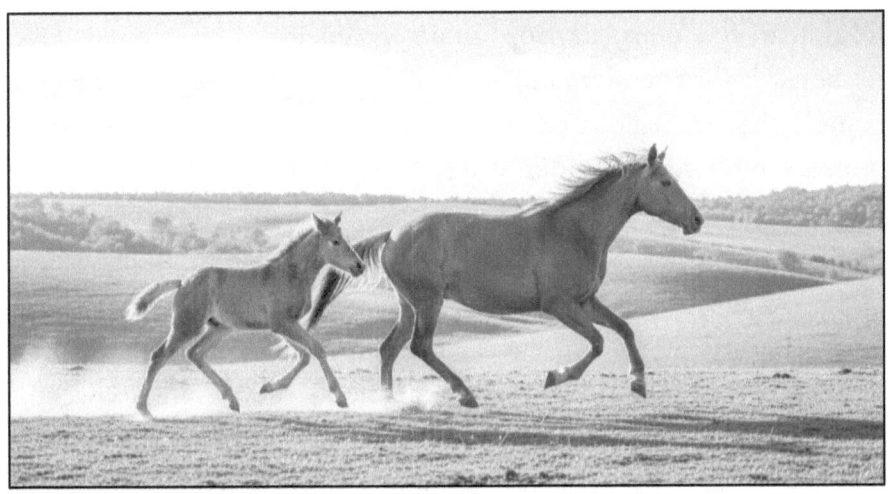

A crucial player in this process is the cerebellum, responsible for refining movement, balance, and coordination. Initially, immature cerebellar connections result in the characteristic jerky movements observed in young foals. However, as myelination progresses, these movements become more fluid and precise. The cerebellum also integrates sensory inputs from the limbs, trunk, and head, allowing for finely tuned locomotion and stability. The **flocculonodular lobe**, a subregion of the cerebellum, processes vestibular information, contributing to balance and spatial orientation, key components of a horse's ability to navigate its environment.

Developmental Sequence and Cognitive Maturation

Myelination occurs in a specific sequence, prioritizing regions essential for survival. The motor roots develop first, followed by sensory pathways and brainstem structures responsible for automatic behaviors and reflexes. This progression allows foals to respond immediately to environmental stimuli, avoiding predators and staying within the protective range of the herd.

While motor and sensory pathways mature early, higher-order cognitive functions develop more gradually. The frontal lobe, responsible for attention, impulse control, and initiating movement, is among the last regions to undergo myelination. As a result, young horses exhibit short attention spans, requiring brief and simple training sessions rather than lengthy, complex ones. Expecting a yearling to maintain focus for extended periods would be akin to asking a third grader to sit through a college-level lecture. Between the ages of two and four, attentional capacity increases, making young horses more capable of sustained attention, comparable to a developing teenager.

The basal ganglia, another key structure, work in tandem with the cerebellum and frontal lobes to refine movement and procedural learning. These subcortical nuclei play a crucial role in habit formation, motor sequencing, and reinforcement learning. As training progresses, well-established motor patterns become more automatic, allowing horses to respond instinctively to cues with minimal cognitive effort.

Neurochemical Influences and White Matter Plasticity

The process of myelination is driven by neurochemical interactions, particularly the role of **glutamate**, the brain's primary excitatory neurotransmitter. Glutamate facilitates communication between neurons and glial cells, promoting the production of myelin. Research in both humans and animals has demonstrated that repeated motor activities enhance white matter density in functionally relevant brain regions. For example, studies in children learning to play the piano have shown increased myelination in areas associated with fine motor control. Similarly, in horses, repeated movements, whether through training or natural locomotion, lead to structural changes that enhance neural efficiency and motor precision.

Moreover, **oligodendrocytes** can dynamically adjust the thickness of myelin sheaths, fine-tuning conduction velocity in response to experience. This adaptability ensures that frequently used neural circuits remain optimized for performance. Training that involves repeated physical movements not only strengthens these pathways but also induces long-term modifications in brain architecture, supporting the horse's ability to learn new skills and refine existing behaviors.

Lifelong Myelination and Neural Adaptability

Although myelination is most rapid in early life, it does not cease in adulthood. The equine brain remains plastic, meaning it continues to adapt based on experience, learning, and environmental interactions. Neural pathways can strengthen, weaken, or even reorganize depending on the demands placed upon them. This plasticity is particularly relevant in training, where repeated exposure to specific cues and motor tasks refines neural connectivity.

Understanding the progression of myelination and its relationship to behavior and learning provides valuable insight into age-appropriate training strategies. Rather than imposing intensive training on a developing horse, handlers can optimize learning by aligning their methods with the horse's neurological capabilities at different life stages. By acknowledging the biological underpinnings of neurodevelopment, we can create training programs that enhance performance while prioritizing equine welfare.

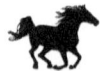

Neuroplasticity

"Neuroplasticity reminds us: no one is ever truly stuck—not the horse, not the rider. Change is written in the synapse."

—Dr. Stephen Peters

Neurons: The Foundation of Brain Function

The horse's brain functions through a sophisticated network of **neurons** that communicate using electrochemical signals. **Neurons**, the fundamental units of the nervous system, consist of three primary components: the **cell body**, **dendrites**, and an **axon**. The **dendrites** act as receivers, collecting incoming signals from other **neurons**, while the **axon** serves as a transmitter, sending these signals to target cells, such as other **neurons**, muscles, or glands.

Neuronal signaling is a dynamic process in which electrochemical messages traverse vast networks, shaping cognition, behavior, and adaptation. **Neurotransmitters**, chemical messengers, bridge the **synaptic** gaps between **neurons**, allowing signals to propagate. The brain is constantly shaping and reconfiguring its **neural architecture** in response to experience. This continuous adaptation ensures that learning, memory, and skill development are always evolving. Importantly, all learning is based on prior learning, as new knowledge and behaviors build upon existing **neural networks** and previously acquired information.

Physical activity, environmental enrichment, problem-solving, and learning tasks enhance the growth and connectivity of **neurons**. Conversely, **stress**, certain types of inflammation, and sensory deprivation can have deleterious effects, leading to the loss of neuronal connections. Isolated **neurons** that fail to receive sufficient input may undergo **pruning**, where inactive connections are eliminated. If **neurons** are alive and active, it is because they participate in some **network**, reinforcing the idea that learning is a dynamic and ongoing process that shapes **neural architecture**.

Any change in knowledge stems from modifications in neuronal networks. Neurons self-modify based on experience, a process central to learning and adaptation. Much of learning involves associating one thing with another, requiring changes in neural connectivity to form new associations. The strength of connections between neurons evolves through experience, allowing the brain to optimize and refine its functions in response to external demands. This adaptability underscores the remarkable plasticity of the equine brain, offering insights into how horses process, retain, and apply information throughout their lives.

Neuroplasticity: The Adaptable Brain

The horse's brain is continuously changing throughout life. This capacity for change, known as neuroplasticity, enables horses to learn from their environment and respond effectively to challenges based on past experiences. At the core of these changes are electrochemical signals that drive every equine thought, reaction, movement, and feeling. These signals travel through a network of nerve fibers, where their strength, speed, and accuracy are enhanced by myelin. The more frequently a particular neural circuit is used, the more it is myelinated by oligodendrocytes, leading to stronger, faster, and more fluent neural activity.

This process has profound implications for training and behavior. Once a circuit is myelinated, it is highly stable, which is why old habits and behaviors are often difficult to break. Creating new circuits requires neglecting old pathways while stimulating new ones through deliberate practice. Early in this process, precision is critical, as myelin formation is highly responsive to accuracy. Repeatedly firing a signal, correcting errors, and refining the circuit strengthens the desired connections and myelination. Furthermore, because all learning builds upon prior experiences, new training efforts must acknowledge and integrate previous conditioning to be effective.

Optimizing Training for Neuroplasticity

The way we train the brain determines how effectively it functions. Clear, precise communication is essential for building accurate neural circuits. Confusion triggers sympathetic arousal (stress responses) that can hinder learning. To construct new pathways, training should involve **"deep practice,"** a process of working just beyond the comfort zone, reflecting on errors, adjusting, and repeating until the desired skill is mastered. Repetition is vital for stimulating myelination. Breaking tasks into small, manageable steps- **"chunking"** -allows for gradual mastery, which can later be integrated into more complex movements.

Repetition plays a crucial role in learning by reinforcing neural pathways, allowing the horse to develop consistency and predictability in its responses. However, excessive repetition, often referred to as drilling, can become counterproductive. While initial repetitions may provide a strong dopamine reinforcement, signaling motivation and reward, each successive repetition tends to yield diminishing returns. As the task becomes overly predictable, dopamine release declines, reducing engagement and enthusiasm. If training persists beyond the horse's optimal learning bracket, the animal may disengage entirely, displaying signs of boredom, frustration, or even learned helplessness. This state, sometimes described as the horse "checking out," occurs when the nervous system no longer finds value or novelty in the experience. Instead of fostering learning, excessive drilling can suppress motivation and hinder retention. Effective training balances structured repetition with variability and rest, ensuring that the horse remains mentally engaged and receptive to learning.

Over time, as skill improves, the brain transitions activity from resource-intensive regions like the frontal lobe to more automatic-processing areas like the basal ganglia. This shift conserves energy and increases efficiency. Unnecessary neural connections are pruned, leaving only the pathways required for streamlined performance.

The Brain's Capacity for Learning

Experience shapes the brain's structure and function. When signals fire repeatedly along axons, the connections between neurons are strengthened, making them easier to activate in the future. Neighboring oligodendrocytes detect these patterns of activity and respond by wrapping myelin around the active circuits, reinforcing the pathways essential for learning.

The brain is fundamentally experience-driven, integrating new information into existing networks. Novices, with fewer prior connections, often struggle to incorporate isolated new information. Without repeated practice and integration, unused information is dropped from the neural network. Dendritic arborization, the sprouting of new nerve fiber branches, allows for greater communication between neurons. Stimulated and engaged neurons develop extensive dendrites, while those with limited stimulation remain sparse, reducing their capacity for communication.

Avoiding Myelination of Errors

Clear, deliberate signals are critical during training. Failing to identify and correct errors allows the horse to myelinate incorrect pathways, strengthening unwanted behaviors. In effect, repetition of errors makes the horse better at performing the error. Thus, trainers must be vigilant in detecting mistakes and guiding the horse toward the wanted correct behavior.

Hebb's Rule and Neuroplasticity

Hebb's Rule encapsulates the foundation of neuroplasticity: **"Neurons that fire together wire together."** Each time an impulse crosses a synapse, it becomes easier for subsequent impulses to do the same. This principle underlies learning and habit formation, highlighting the importance of consistency and precision in practice.

Practical Implications

Spaced Learning: Slower, spaced-out learning promotes greater neuroplasticity and long-term retention compared to rapid, massed learning.

Energy Conservation: Conscious processing requires more energy than unconscious, automatic processes. Neuroplasticity enables the nervous system to shift learned behaviors to unconscious control, conserving energy while maintaining efficiency.

Integration: Over time, neural changes integrate new experiences into a vast associative network, allowing advanced learners to process complex information more efficiently.

The brain's ability to change through experience underscores the importance of intentional, well-structured training. Precision, patience, and repetition drive myelin formation, enhancing both physical and cognitive performance. By understanding and leveraging neuroplasticity, we can optimize learning and promote lasting, positive change in equine behavior and skill development.

With the basics of brain structure and adaptability established, we now turn our attention to the intricate biochemical forces that modulate neural function. The nervous system does not operate in isolation; rather, it engages in a dynamic interplay with hormones and neurotransmitters, chemical messengers that modulate and fine-tune cognition, emotion, and behavior. These molecular signals orchestrate everything from emotional regulation and stress responses to learning and memory, shaping how horses perceive and interact with their environment. By exploring the neuroendocrine system, we will gain deeper insight into how internal states influence external actions, laying the foundation for a more nuanced understanding of equine behavior.

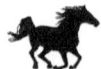

Neuroendocrinology

Equine neuroendocrinology explores the integration of the nervous and endocrine systems, highlighting their coordinated roles in regulating physiological processes and behavior. At the heart of this integration are chemical messengers—including hormones, neuropeptides, neurotransmitters, and neuromodulators—that communicate across neural and endocrine pathways. These molecules modulate a broad range of equine functions, such as metabolism, growth, stress responses, emotional states, learning, social interactions, and reproductive behaviors. Hormonal signals can originate centrally, through the brain's hypothalamus and pituitary gland, or peripherally from glands such as the adrenals. Both neural and hormonal signals can produce immediate responses or initiate sustained physiological changes, enabling horses to effectively adapt to internal demands and external environmental conditions. This chapter details the essential roles these neuroendocrine messengers play in equine biology, providing the scientific basis needed to understand their influence on behavior, training outcomes, and overall welfare.

Oxytocin is a neuropeptide synthesized in the paraventricular and supraoptic nuclei of the hypothalamus and released into systemic circulation via the posterior pituitary gland. In addition to its peripheral effects, oxytocin exerts central neuromodulatory influence on brain systems involved in emotional regulation, social cognition, and affiliative behavior. One of its primary anxiolytic mechanisms involves dampening activity in the lateral central nucleus of the amygdala, a region critical for processing threat and fear-related stimuli. Concurrently, oxytocin interacts with mesolimbic reward pathways by binding to receptors in the ventral striatum, facilitating dopamine release and reinforcing social bonding through mechanisms of positive reinforcement.

In the equine brain, the oxytocinergic system supports essential social behaviors including maternal care, pair bonding, mutual grooming, and herd cohesion. Affiliative interactions such as synchronized grooming or gentle physical contact result in measurable increases in circulating oxytocin, reduced sympathetic arousal, and improved emotional regulation. These neurochemically reinforced behaviors contribute to herd stability, strengthen social hierarchies, and promote behavioral flexibility. Conversely, social disruption—such as prolonged isolation, abrupt separation, or inconsistent handling—can suppress oxytocin release, elevate hypothalamic-pituitary-adrenal (HPA) axis activation, and increase anxiety, vigilance, and behavioral reactivity.

From a neurobehavioral perspective, oxytocin facilitates social learning by enhancing the salience of affiliative cues and improving attentional focus in emotionally secure contexts. When training is conducted within environments that promote safety, predictability, and relational consistency, conditions are optimized for oxytocin release and reinforcement-based learning. This biochemical state supports more effective acquisition, memory consolidation, and long-term behavioral change.

Clinically, oxytocin functions at the intersection of stress modulation, reward processing, and social affiliation. Understanding its role in the equine nervous system provides a mechanistic foundation for ethical horsemanship practices that prioritize emotional safety and relational integrity. By engaging the oxytocinergic system, horse–human interactions can support not only behavioral outcomes but also welfare and resilience across a range of contexts—from foundational handling to high-performance training and therapeutic applications.

The Vasopressin–Testosterone Axis in Stallions

Vasopressin is a neuropeptide closely related to oxytocin; both evolved from a shared ancestral molecule called **vasotocin**, and both play key roles in modulating social behavior. Vasopressin is synthesized in the hypothalamus and released through the posterior pituitary, where it exerts systemic physiological effects such as regulating blood pressure and water balance. However, its influence extends far beyond homeostasis, particularly in the social dynamics of the equine brain.

In horses—and especially in stallions—vasopressin contributes to behaviors associated with social vigilance, territoriality, and defensive aggression. It heightens alertness and reactive behavior during competitive or stressful social situations, reinforcing dominance hierarchies that promote herd cohesion and reproductive success. While oxytocin is more associated with bonding and safety, vasopressin supports bonding through protection and boundary-setting—functions especially critical in male social roles.

The behavioral effects of vasopressin are significantly amplified by testosterone, which acts as a neuromodulatory enhancer. Testosterone increases vasopressin production and upregulates vasopressin receptor density, particularly V1a receptors in key brain areas such as the hypothalamus, amygdala, septum, and bed nucleus of the stria terminalis (BNST). This interaction forms a powerful neuroendocrine axis that drives many behaviors traditionally associated with masculinity: territorial defense, mate guarding, protective vigilance, and social competition.

This axis is particularly active in breeding contexts or in the presence of rival males and mares—circumstances where dominance, access, and status are contested. It enables stallions to respond swiftly and assertively to social challenges, with vasopressin as the molecular signaler and testosterone as the volume control.

Understanding this interaction allows for a more sophisticated view of stallion behavior. Rather than relying on simplistic or anthropomorphic labels like "aggressive" or "dominant," we can recognize these behaviors as neurobiologically mediated adaptations—and shape management strategies that respect both the horse's welfare and the intricacies of its brain.

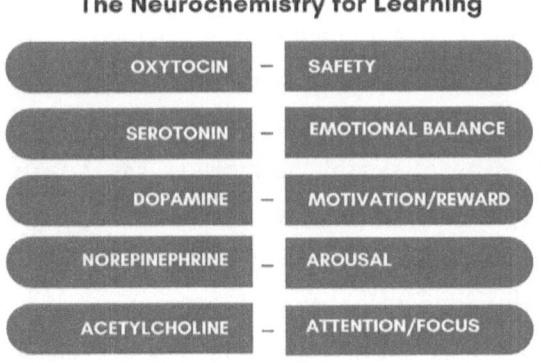

Dopamine is a catecholamine neurotransmitter that plays a fundamental role in the regulation of motivation, reward processing, goal-directed behavior, and motor control in the equine brain. Synthesized primarily in dopaminergic neurons of the ventral tegmental area (VTA) and the substantia nigra pars compacta, dopamine acts through multiple projection pathways, including the mesolimbic, mesocortical, and nigrostriatal systems. These pathways support a wide range of functions—from initiating voluntary movement to reinforcing behavioral learning and shaping attentional focus.

Within the mesolimbic system, dopaminergic projections from the VTA to the nucleus accumbens underlie the neurobiology of incentive salience—how horses assign value to stimuli and direct behavior toward obtaining rewards. This circuitry becomes particularly active in response to reward anticipation, novelty, or unexpected positive outcomes. In equine training contexts, dopamine is released in response to cues associated with relief from pressure, food rewards, and pleasurable social or sensory interactions. The reinforcing properties of timely, well-structured training are largely mediated by this dopaminergic activity, making it a central mechanism in both operant and classical conditioning.

The motivational salience encoded by dopamine is not limited to primary rewards. Horses, like other mammals, exhibit dopaminergic responses to novelty and uncertainty—elements that can increase exploratory behavior and engagement. This suggests that varying the training environment, introducing mild novelty, and maintaining predictability within a flexible framework can enhance learning by stimulating dopaminergic pathways. In contrast, excessive repetition, monotony, or poorly timed cues may lead to diminished dopaminergic activity, a reduction in behavioral responsiveness, and decreased learning efficacy. This habituation effect is a neurochemical reflection of declining motivational drive in the absence of meaningful reinforcement or variation.

Beyond the mesolimbic system, dopamine synthesized in the substantia nigra is crucial for motor function, projecting via the nigrostriatal pathway to the dorsal striatum. This circuit regulates voluntary movement, motor precision, and initiation. Deficits in this system in other species, including humans, are associated with bradykinesia and motor rigidity, as seen in Parkinsonian syndromes. Although such neurodegenerative disorders are not typically described in equine populations, the role of dopamine in coordinating movement remains essential, particularly in performance horses where motor control and motivational state must be finely tuned.

Dopamine also interfaces with learning systems via the mesocortical pathway, projecting to regions of the prefrontal cortex involved in executive function, working memory, and decision-making. This contributes to behavioral flexibility, task persistence, and the ability to evaluate outcomes relative to expectations—core elements of adaptive learning and training retention.

From a practical standpoint, ethical horsemanship that utilizes timely pressure-and-release techniques, clear reinforcement patterns, and appropriately varied training environments directly engages dopaminergic systems to support learning and engagement. Creating opportunities for the horse to "solve problems" and earn reward through cooperation fosters intrinsic motivation and reduces the likelihood of apathy or resistance.

Dopamine, therefore, is not simply a chemical of pleasure or movement—it is a neurobiological engine for motivation, expectation, and learning. Its careful engagement is central to effective, humane training approaches that build attentiveness, curiosity, and behavioral resilience in the horse.

Serotonin (5-hydroxytryptamine, or 5-HT) is a monoamine neurotransmitter synthesized primarily in the raphe nuclei of the brainstem, with an estimated 90–95% of total serotonin produced peripherally in the gastrointestinal tract, specifically within enterochromaffin cells of the intestinal mucosa. Though central and peripheral serotonin are functionally distinct—separated by the blood–brain barrier—both contribute to homeostatic regulation, behavioral modulation, and systemic stress resilience. In the equine nervous system, central serotonin functions as a key modulator of emotional tone, behavioral flexibility, and environmental adaptability.

Centrally, serotonergic neurons originating in the dorsal and median raphe nuclei project widely throughout the brain, influencing regions involved in affective regulation, such as the amygdala, hippocampus, prefrontal cortex, and hypothalamus. Through these projections, serotonin plays a central role in modulating threat responses, behavioral inhibition, emotional reactivity, and neuroplastic adaptation to stress. Adequate serotonergic tone is associated with emotional stability, calm attentiveness, and behavioral flexibility—all characteristics conducive to learning, relational engagement, and resilience in the face of environmental challenges.

In horses, a well-regulated serotonin system supports the ability to remain composed and behaviorally responsive rather than reactive. This neurochemical balance enhances the horse's capacity to process social cues, tolerate frustration, and recover from startling or aversive stimuli. In contrast, dysregulated or reduced central serotonin transmission has been linked to increased irritability, impulsivity, aggression, stereotypic behaviors (e.g., cribbing, weaving), and a diminished threshold for stress-related responses. These patterns mirror findings in other mammalian species and underscore serotonin's essential role in behavioral regulation and welfare.

Peripherally, serotonin influences gastrointestinal motility, immune signaling, and the gut–brain axis—a bidirectional communication network increasingly recognized as integral to affective regulation. Though peripheral serotonin does not cross into the brain, its role in gut health, vagal tone, and inflammatory signaling may indirectly influence central emotional states. Disruptions in the gut microbiome, chronic stress, or poor nutrition may alter serotonin metabolism and impact both gastrointestinal and neurobehavioral health.

Understanding serotonin's neurobehavioral role highlights the importance of creating calm, enriched environments that minimize unpredictable stressors and support behavioral regulation. Training protocols that avoid chronic activation of the sympathetic nervous system, respect thresholds, and promote consistency can help stabilize serotonergic tone. Additionally, attention to nutritional health, gut function, and overall welfare may support peripheral pathways that influence central affective states.

Serotonin, therefore, is not merely a "mood chemical"—it is a neuromodulatory regulator of safety, impulse control, and adaptability. Its influence extends across systems and timescales, shaping how horses perceive, respond to, and recover from the demands of their environment.

Norepinephrine (NE), also known as noradrenaline, is a catecholamine neurotransmitter and neuromodulator produced primarily by neurons in the locus coeruleus, a compact nucleus located in the dorsal pons of the brainstem. The locus coeruleus is the principal site of norepinephrine synthesis in the central nervous system and exerts widespread influence through its extensive projections to the cerebral cortex, hippocampus, amygdala, thalamus, hypothalamus, cerebellum, and spinal cord. This system plays a fundamental role in initiating and regulating arousal, vigilance, and rapid responsiveness to environmental change.

In the horse, the norepinephrine system is activated in response to novelty, uncertainty, or perceived threat. Upon activation, norepinephrine is rapidly released into target brain regions and peripheral tissues, producing a cascade of physiological effects: heightened sensory acuity, increased heart rate, pupil dilation, elevated muscle tone, and a general state of somatic readiness. This acute state of arousal facilitates immediate action—an adaptive feature central to survival in prey species whose evolutionary success depends on rapid detection and response to external cues.

The functional role of norepinephrine is tightly coupled with the dynamics of the autonomic nervous system. It is a key driver of sympathetic activation, preparing the body for "fight or flight" responses. This neural activity is often paralleled and sustained by the slower-acting endocrine release of glucocorticoids—most notably cortisol—from the adrenal cortex. While norepinephrine facilitates immediate mobilization and sensory prioritization, glucocorticoids support extended metabolic demands by enhancing energy availability, modulating inflammation, and influencing longer-term behavioral adaptations.

Importantly, the balance and duration of norepinephrine release determine whether arousal remains adaptive or becomes maladaptive. Short bursts of norepinephrine facilitate focused attention, learning, and appropriate behavioral reactivity. However, chronic or excessive norepinephrine activity—whether from repeated environmental stressors, poorly timed training stimuli, or inconsistent handling—can lead to hypervigilance, anxiety, reduced learning efficiency, and difficulty in behavioral regulation. Overactivation of this system is also associated with sleep disruption, heightened startle reflexes, and persistent autonomic dysregulation.

In equine behavior and training, an understanding of norepinephrine's role is essential for interpreting arousal states and modulating engagement strategies. Training that escalates sympathetic tone without allowing for recovery can result in sensitization rather than habituation. Conversely, practices that promote a return to parasympathetic dominance—such as rhythmic touch, breath regulation in the handler, or structured routines with clear cues—can help restore autonomic balance and support learning.

The locus coeruleus–norepinephrine system operates as an internal alerting network—modulating salience, prioritizing threats, and allocating cognitive resources. When appropriately engaged, it facilitates attention, memory encoding, and behavioral flexibility. When overdriven, it contributes to dysregulation and emotional reactivity. Evidence-based practices that attune to these neurophysiological dynamics can better support a horse's ability to remain alert without becoming overwhelmed, enhancing both welfare and performance.

Acetylcholine is one of the most important neuromodulators in the equine nervous system, playing a central role in attention, learning, memory, and physiological regulation. In the horse's brain, a key source of acetylcholine is the **nucleus basalis of Meynert**, located in the basal forebrain. This structure sends widespread cholinergic projections throughout the cerebral cortex, modulating cortical activity during states of focused attention. When a horse is alert and engaged, acetylcholine is released in a way that enhances the signal-to-noise ratio in cortical circuits. This means that relevant sensory input is amplified, while irrelevant background activity is suppressed. In practical terms, this neurochemical process enables the horse to filter distractions and attend to specific cues from the environment or handler—an ability that is essential not only for survival in the wild but also for effective learning in training environments.

Beyond modulating attention, acetylcholine plays a crucial role in learning and memory formation. During the acquisition of new skills or information, acetylcholine helps "tag" active neural pathways, marking them for **synaptic strengthening** through a process known as long-term potentiation (LTP). This synaptic tagging supports the formation of durable neural connections that encode learned behaviors and patterns. In a training context, when a horse is calm, attentive, and repeatedly engaged with a well-timed cue or task, acetylcholine facilitates the encoding of that experience into memory. However, if the horse is in a state of stress, distraction, or hyperarousal, the effectiveness of cholinergic signaling is diminished, impairing attention and learning. This underscores the importance of emotional regulation and an appropriate learning environment.

Acetylcholine is also deeply involved in regulating sleep–wake cycles and plays a pivotal role in REM sleep, a phase essential for memory consolidation. In horses, as in humans, sleep is not merely a rest state but a critical period during which the brain replays and integrates the day's learning experiences. Acetylcholine levels increase during REM sleep, supporting this integration process. Without adequate sleep—particularly REM and slow-wave stages—the consolidation of new learning is compromised.

In essence, acetylcholine acts as a kind of neurobiological spotlight, illuminating the circuits of attention, tagging new experiences for long-term memory, and orchestrating internal states that support optimal learning.

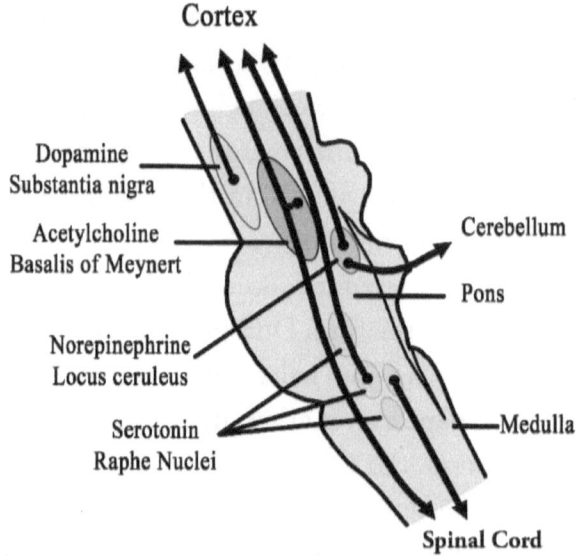

Glucocorticoids, primarily **cortisol** in horses, are steroid hormones released from the adrenal cortex in response to activation of the hypothalamic-pituitary-adrenal (HPA) axis. Cortisol plays a central role in the physiological adaptation to stress, working in tandem with fast-acting catecholamines such as norepinephrine to support both immediate and sustained responses to perceived threat or environmental challenge. While norepinephrine initiates acute arousal, cortisol mobilizes metabolic resources to sustain activity, regulate inflammation, and restore homeostasis once the immediate threat has passed.

In the short term, cortisol release is adaptive. It enhances glucose availability by promoting gluconeogenesis, redirects energy toward essential survival systems, and supports cardiovascular and cognitive function during heightened demand. This enables the horse to maintain alertness and physical readiness beyond the initial sympathetic activation window. However, the same properties that make cortisol beneficial in acute contexts can become harmful when elevation is chronic or dysregulated.

Prolonged cortisol exposure, often resulting from chronic stress, social instability, overtraining, or inadequate recovery, can impair multiple systems. Sustained glucocorticoid elevation has been shown to reduce neurogenesis in the hippocampus, a brain region critical for learning and memory. It can also lead to dendritic atrophy, synaptic loss, and suppression of brain-derived neurotrophic factor (BDNF), thereby compromising neural plasticity and adaptive learning. Systemically, chronic cortisol suppresses immune function, disrupts sleep patterns, and contributes to metabolic dysfunction—factors that can negatively impact both performance and welfare in horses.

Importantly, the sensitivity and regulation of the HPA axis are shaped early in life. Maternal care, social buffering, and early environmental stability influence the expression and distribution of glucocorticoid receptors in limbic structures such as the hippocampus and amygdala. These epigenetic effects play a key role in determining the individual's lifelong stress responsivity and emotional resilience. Horses that experience consistent, nurturing early-life interactions tend to develop more efficient HPA axis feedback mechanisms, enabling quicker recovery from stress and greater behavioral adaptability. In contrast, horses raised under inconsistent, neglectful, or aversive conditions may exhibit hypersensitive stress systems, reduced coping capacity, and heightened baseline cortisol levels.

From a horsemanship perspective, monitoring and managing cumulative stress load is essential. Practices that allow for predictability, rest, social contact, and a gradual escalation of training demands help regulate cortisol levels and prevent maladaptive stress states. Conversely, abrupt transitions, social isolation, excessive physical exertion without recovery, or prolonged exposure to ambiguous or aversive cues can push the HPA axis toward chronic activation, increasing the risk of behavioral dysregulation and physical illness.

Cortisol is not inherently harmful; it is a vital hormone for adaptation and survival. However, the frequency, duration, and context of its activation determine whether it promotes resilience or contributes to vulnerability. Ethical, neuroscience-informed horsemanship involves not only recognizing visible signs of stress but also understanding the underlying neuroendocrine mechanisms that shape the horse's internal experience across time.

Glutamate is the primary excitatory neurotransmitter in the mammalian central nervous system and plays a fundamental role in synaptic transmission, neural plasticity, and experience-dependent learning. In the equine brain, glutamate is central to processes that enable adaptation, memory consolidation, motor coordination, and behavioral flexibility—key attributes in both natural survival and the applied context of horsemanship and training.

Glutamate exerts its effects by binding to several classes of postsynaptic receptors, most notably the ionotropic NMDA (N-methyl-D-aspartate) and AMPA (α-amino-3-hydroxy-5-methyl-4-isoxazolepropionic acid) receptors. Activation of NMDA receptors is particularly significant for initiating **long-term potentiation (LTP)**, a synaptic mechanism whereby repeated stimulation strengthens communication between neurons. LTP is widely recognized as a cellular basis for learning and memory. In horses, as in other species, this synaptic reinforcement enables the consolidation of conditioned responses, shaping how sensory cues, motor patterns, and emotional states become encoded through repetition and experience.

Beyond synaptic plasticity, glutamate supports myelination and facilitates the development of interconnected neural networks by influencing oligodendrocyte activity and neuron–glia communication. These processes are critical for efficient signal transmission across brain regions, underpinning the refinement of motor skills, sensorimotor integration, and complex coordination—capacities especially relevant in young, developing horses or those undergoing intensive physical training.

Importantly, glutamate does not act in isolation. It functions within a highly interactive neurochemical environment, dynamically modulating and being modulated by systems including dopamine (motivation and reward), acetylcholine (attention and learning), and cortisol (stress regulation). This neurochemical interplay affects how horses process novelty, attend to environmental stimuli, and encode experience. For example, in the context of training, novelty-driven dopaminergic signals may heighten glutamatergic plasticity, enhancing learning when paired with rewarding or emotionally salient outcomes. Conversely, high levels of cortisol from chronic stress can dysregulate glutamate signaling, potentially impairing synaptic function and reducing learning capacity.

While glutamate is essential for neuroplasticity, excessive or dysregulated glutamatergic activity can be neurotoxic, particularly under conditions of sustained stress, trauma, or metabolic dysfunction. Prolonged glutamate elevation can lead to excitotoxicity—overactivation of NMDA receptors resulting in calcium influx, oxidative stress, and neuronal injury. This underscores the importance of balanced arousal and recovery in training and management protocols.

From a practical standpoint, ethical horsemanship that emphasizes timing, consistency, and appropriate repetition engages glutamatergic mechanisms to support adaptive neural remodeling. Structured learning environments that offer clear cues, rest intervals, and variability within a predictable framework optimize synaptic efficiency and reduce the risk of overstimulation. By aligning with the principles of experience-dependent plasticity, trainers can shape the equine brain in ways that foster lasting learning while minimizing the potential for stress-induced maladaptation.

In sum, glutamate is the engine of neuroplastic change. It encodes experience at the cellular level, builds and maintains communication pathways, and integrates the horse's perception, movement, and memory into coherent behavioral responses.

Gamma-aminobutyric acid (GABA) is the principal inhibitory neurotransmitter in the equine central nervous system and plays a critical role in maintaining neural homeostasis by counterbalancing excitatory signals—particularly those mediated by glutamate. GABAergic signaling is essential for regulating arousal, emotional reactivity, motor control, and the modulation of stress responses. It functions as a neurochemical "braking system," enabling the nervous system to filter and fine-tune responses to both internal and external stimuli.

GABA operates primarily through two receptor types: **GABA-A**, a ligand-gated chloride channel responsible for fast synaptic inhibition, and **GABA-B**, a G-protein-coupled receptor involved in slower, longer-lasting inhibitory effects. Binding of GABA to these receptors leads to neuronal hyperpolarization and a decreased likelihood of action potential generation. This inhibitory action shapes the timing, amplitude, and spread of neural activity, preventing excessive excitation that could otherwise result in dysregulation, anxiety, or impaired learning.

In the equine limbic system—particularly in regions such as the amygdala and hippocampus—GABAergic neurons modulate emotional intensity and behavioral responses to stress. By dampening overactivation in these areas, GABA promotes emotional stability, reduces hypervigilance, and fosters conditions conducive to social bonding and trust-building. These mechanisms are particularly relevant during training, where emotional overload or inconsistent pressure can overwhelm the horse's capacity to learn and regulate behavior. A well-regulated GABA system allows for calmer engagement, improved attentional control, and a reduction in startle or escape behaviors.

GABA also exerts regulatory control over the **hypothalamic-pituitary-adrenal (HPA) axis**, modulating the neuroendocrine cascade that governs the stress response. Inhibitory GABAergic inputs to the hypothalamus help suppress excessive release of corticotropin-releasing hormone (CRH), which in turn reduces downstream production of adrenocorticotropic hormone (ACTH) and cortisol. This top-down inhibition provides a buffering effect against chronic stress, supporting resilience and reducing the risk of long-term maladaptive changes in brain structure and function.

In addition to its role in emotional regulation, GABA is a key modulator of the **sleep–wake cycle**, particularly in the initiation and maintenance of slow-wave (non-REM) sleep. Sleep, in turn, is critical for memory consolidation, synaptic pruning, and motor learning. During rest, GABA-mediated inhibition allows the nervous system to downregulate sympathetic tone, integrate newly formed neural circuits, and refine sensorimotor coordination. Horses deprived of adequate sleep—whether due to environmental disruption, pain, or chronic stress—may show signs of irritability, impaired learning, and increased reactivity, reflecting underlying disruptions in GABAergic regulation.

From a training and welfare standpoint, environments that are perceived as safe, predictable, and non-threatening enhance GABAergic tone and promote conditions for learning and behavioral plasticity. Conversely, excessive stimulation, inconsistency, or lack of recovery time can suppress GABA function, shift the brain toward excitatory dominance, and impair both cognitive and emotional regulation. Training strategies that respect thresholds, incorporate calm transitions, and prioritize emotional containment actively engage GABAergic mechanisms to support successful outcomes.

In essence, GABA serves as the neurobiological counterweight to arousal and excitation. Its inhibitory actions are not passive; they are actively involved in shaping perception, regulating behavior, and maintaining physiological balance. By facilitating calm engagement and emotional composure, GABA enables the horse's brain to remain in a state conducive to learning, adaptation, and relational trust.

Brain-Derived Neurotrophic Factor (BDNF) is a critical neurotrophin that supports neuronal survival, synaptic modulation, and adaptive neuroplasticity. In the equine brain, BDNF facilitates the dynamic remodeling of neural networks in response to learning, environmental input, and stress exposure. Its actions are mediated through high-affinity binding to the TrkB (tropomyosin receptor kinase B) receptor, promoting synaptic efficiency, dendritic growth, and long-term potentiation (LTP) in key regions such as the hippocampus, cortex, and basal forebrain. These mechanisms are foundational to learning, memory consolidation, and behavioral flexibility.

Recent research further identifies the BDNF/TrkB system as playing an inhibitory role in the **oval nucleus of the bed nucleus of the stria terminalis (ovBNST)**—a subregion of the extended amygdala implicated in anxiety regulation and maladaptive stress responses. Within the ovBNST, BDNF/TrkB signaling induces a hyperpolarizing shift in membrane potential via inwardly rectifying potassium currents and promotes long-term depression (LTD) at postsynaptic sites. This synaptic inhibition serves to dampen excitability in stress-sensitive neurons, providing a neurobiological mechanism for buffering fear-related behaviors and recalibrating the system under prolonged stress. This finding reframes BDNF not only as a neuroplastic facilitator but also as a regulatory agent capable of dampening maladaptive reactivity in extended limbic circuits.

In horses, BDNF expression is strongly influenced by physical activity, novelty, social enrichment, and environmental predictability. Aerobic movement and exploratory behaviors naturally elevate BDNF levels, enhancing both synaptic resilience and emotional regulation. Conversely, chronic stress, social isolation, sleep deprivation, and high-cortisol states—often resulting from environmental unpredictability or overtraining—suppress BDNF synthesis and impair plasticity in stress-regulating circuits. Importantly, glucocorticoids such as cortisol antagonize

BDNF transcription, weakening the brain's ability to form adaptive responses to training or environmental change.

Dietary influences also modulate BDNF. Diets high in refined carbohydrates, unhealthy fats, and processed feeds are associated with decreased neurotrophin expression, whereas nutrient-dense diets rich in omega-3 fatty acids, polyphenols, and antioxidants support neural health and BDNF production. Additionally, sleep—particularly the deep stages of slow-wave and REM sleep—facilitates BDNF-dependent memory consolidation and circuit refinement, both of which are essential for motor learning and behavioral adaptation in horses.

From a horsemanship standpoint, training environments that incorporate low-stress exposure, predictable patterns, novelty within a secure framework, and ample physical movement are optimal for engaging BDNF-mediated neuroplasticity. In doing so, they not only facilitate learning but also support recovery from stress and build long-term emotional resilience.

BDNF is thus a multifaceted regulator—promoting growth when the system is in a state of engagement and inhibiting maladaptive activation under conditions of stress. By supporting its expression and regulatory function, we create the neurobiological conditions for horses to thrive cognitively, emotionally, and behaviorally.

Endorphins, short for "endogenous morphine-like substances," are a class of opioid neuropeptides produced primarily in the hypothalamus and pituitary gland. They function as part of the body's intrinsic pain-regulating system, acting on mu-opioid receptors throughout the central nervous system to reduce the perception of pain and modulate affective states. Among them, **beta-endorphin** is the most potent and extensively studied, playing a central role in the horse's physiological and behavioral response to stress, exertion, and injury.

Endorphin release is typically triggered by nociceptive input (pain), prolonged stress, or sustained physical activity. Once released, endorphins inhibit the transmission of pain signals at both spinal and supraspinal levels, producing analgesia and, in some cases, euphoria. This neurochemical effect underlies phenomena such as the "runner's high" and may contribute to the sense of calm or satisfaction horses display after prolonged galloping, rolling, or mutual grooming. In training or athletic contexts, endorphin release can support resilience by blunting discomfort and maintaining engagement despite increasing physical demands.

However, beta-endorphin is also released under conditions of **chronic or inescapable stress**, where its role may shift from acute pain modulation to longer-term affective adaptation. In such states, elevated beta-endorphin may serve as an internal buffer, suppressing the psychological and physiological impacts of distress. While this adaptation can temporarily protect the individual, it also carries important behavioral implications—particularly in environments that restrict movement, social interaction, or sensory stimulation.

A growing body of research suggests that endorphin signaling contributes to the development of stereotypic behaviors in horses— repetitive, once thought to be functionless actions such as cribbing, weaving, and stall walking. These behaviors are frequently observed in horses housed under restrictive or monotonous conditions and are now hypothesized to function as self-soothing mechanisms, partially mediated by endogenous opioid release. In this model, the behavior itself becomes a stimulus for beta-endorphin secretion, establishing a neurochemical feedback loop that reinforces the pattern. While such behaviors may provide transient relief, they also indicate underlying neurobiological dysregulation and compromised welfare.

Importantly, opioid systems interact with other neuromodulatory networks—including dopamine (reward), serotonin (emotional balance), and cortisol (stress adaptation)—further complicating the picture. For example, endorphin-dopamine interactions in the nucleus accumbens may contribute to the reinforcing properties of both natural and maladaptive behaviors. Chronic engagement of these circuits without appropriate environmental modulation can lead to entrenched behavioral patterns that are resistant to extinction.

From a management and training perspective, minimizing the need for compensatory endorphin release is essential. Providing consistent access to movement, social interaction, foraging opportunities, and cognitive engagement reduces reliance on internal coping systems and supports a more balanced neurochemical state. When endorphin-mediated behaviors do arise, they should be interpreted not simply as "bad habits," but as **neuroadaptive responses to environmental inadequacy**—requiring thoughtful intervention at the level of management, enrichment, and relational context.

Endorphins thus occupy a dual role: they are vital for supporting equine endurance, emotional buffering, and pain tolerance, yet their dysregulation may signal compromised welfare. Understanding the context and consequences of endorphin release offers valuable insight into both adaptive and maladaptive responses in horses, emphasizing the importance of designing environments and training protocols that promote neurochemical balance and behavioral health.

Let There Be Light: Equine Light Cycles

The changing seasons and daily cycles of sunlight profoundly influence horse physiology and behavior through intricate **photoneuroendocrine** mechanisms. Central to these processes is the horse's internal master clock, the **suprachiasmatic nucleus (SCN)** of the hypothalamus, which synchronizes internal biological rhythms to external light-dark cycles. Specialized photoreceptive cells in the retina, particularly **intrinsically photosensitive retinal ganglion cells (ipRGCs),** detect ambient light, with heightened sensitivity to blue wavelengths. These cells transmit photic information directly to the SCN via the **retinohypothalamic** tract, allowing horses to entrain their circadian rhythms precisely to environmental conditions.

The SCN regulates the rhythmic secretion of **melatonin** from the **pineal gland**. Melatonin production peaks during darkness and is inhibited by exposure to light, thus reflecting day length through its duration rather than its absolute concentration. Longer winter nights lead to extended melatonin secretion periods, while shorter summer nights produce brief melatonin signals. The duration of melatonin release serves as a robust seasonal cue, enabling the equine brain to track changing seasons accurately.

In reproductively active horses, these melatonin-mediated signals critically influence reproductive timing. Horses, as long-day breeders, respond to lengthening daylight hours in spring and summer with a reduced duration of melatonin secretion. This shortened melatonin signal prompts the hypothalamus to increase the synthesis and release of **gonadotropin-releasing hormone (GnRH)**. GnRH subsequently stimulates the anterior pituitary gland to secrete **luteinizing hormone (LH)** and **follicle-stimulating hormone (FSH)**, triggering ovarian activity and estrous cycles in mares, as well as heightened testosterone production, increased sperm quality, and enhanced sexual behavior in stallions. Conversely, prolonged melatonin secretion during the shorter days of fall and winter suppresses this reproductive cascade, leading mares into anestrus and diminishing libido and fertility in stallions.

Beyond reproduction, melatonin interacts extensively with critical neurotransmitter systems such as serotonin and dopamine, which govern emotional balance, mood regulation, and motivation. Seasonal fluctuations in melatonin levels can thus lead to subtle changes in horse temperament, arousal levels, social behaviors, and cognitive performance. Some horses may exhibit increased anxiety, withdrawal, or excitability depending on their individual sensitivity to these neurochemical shifts. Additionally, melatonin's antioxidant properties provide protective effects against oxidative stress, supporting immune function, neuronal health, and potentially modulating pain sensitivity.

The influence of the SCN extends further through interactions with other hypothalamic nuclei that regulate appetite, metabolic rate, thermoregulation, and the autonomic nervous system. Consequently, seasonal changes in photoperiod may alter feeding behavior, energy metabolism, and physiological stress responses. Neurotransmitters like norepinephrine, which modulates arousal and vigilance, and acetylcholine, critical for attention, are also rhythmically influenced by daylight exposure.

In practical equine management, understanding these photoneuroendocrine relationships is invaluable. For example, artificial lighting regimens of approximately 16 hours of daily illumination for 60 to 90 days effectively simulate spring-like conditions, accelerating the onset of estrous cycles in mares. Awareness of seasonal hormonal fluctuations can also guide stallion handling and training strategies, mitigating heightened aggression and arousal observed during springtime peaks in testosterone. Even non-breeding horses, including geldings and non-reproductive mares, may display seasonal variations in reactivity and motivation, driven by these underlying neurological and endocrine mechanisms.

Sunlight is an influential environmental regulator intricately linked to the equine nervous and endocrine systems. The dynamic interplay between retinal photoreception, SCN-mediated circadian control, melatonin signaling, and downstream hormonal pathways allows horses to adapt seamlessly to seasonal variations.

Equine Cushing's Disease (PPID)

While this book is not intended as a veterinary text, a brief discussion of **Pituitary Pars Intermedia Dysfunction (PPID)**—commonly known as equine Cushing's disease—offers a striking example of how disruptions in the neuroendocrine system can profoundly affect both physiology and behavior. PPID is fundamentally a disorder of dopaminergic regulation within the hypothalamus, specifically targeting the pars intermedia of the pituitary gland. In healthy horses, dopaminergic neurons originating in the hypothalamus exert inhibitory control over this region, thereby regulating the release of several hormones. With advancing age or neurodegeneration, this dopamine-mediated inhibition diminishes. As a result, the **pars intermedia** undergoes hypertrophy and becomes hyperactive, leading to excessive secretion of hormones such as **ACTH (adrenocorticotropic hormone)**. Elevated ACTH, in turn, stimulates the adrenal glands to produce higher levels of cortisol—a glucocorticoid that plays a central role in stress response, metabolism, and immune modulation. Chronic dysregulation of cortisol can contribute to many of the systemic signs seen in PPID, including insulin resistance, muscle wasting, altered fat distribution, abnormal hair growth (hirsutism), lethargy, and a general decline in vitality. These physiological changes can manifest behaviorally, influencing the horse's responsiveness, reactivity, and trainability. From a neuroscience perspective, PPID vividly illustrates how loss of dopaminergic tone in the aging brain initiates a cascade of endocrine changes with far-reaching consequences. This neurodegenerative process bears striking parallels to human conditions such as Parkinson's disease, where dopamine loss similarly leads to impairments in motor control, cognitive function, and hormonal regulation. For horse owners and trainers, understanding PPID as a neuroendocrine disorder of the aging brain—rather than merely a hormonal imbalance—provides critical insight into the complex interplay between brain chemistry, physiology, and behavior in the aging horse.

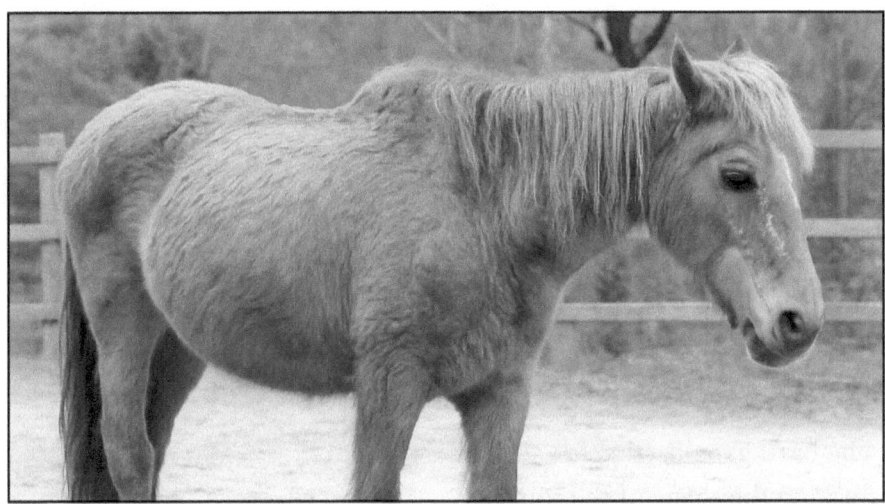

"The Dopamine Drift"
by Dr. Stephen Peters

It begins before the cue—
in the lean of the body,
the flick of an ear,
the moment you both wonder
what might happen next.

Not demand,
but discovery.

The basal ganglia stirs,
tracking the shape of the routine.
Patterns form.
Expectations hum.

And there it is—
a try,
barely more than a shift of weight,
a question asked with the body.

You release.
Timing perfect.
Pressure melts like snow.

And somewhere deep in the midbrain,
dopamine rises—
not in triumph,
but in affirmation.

Yes.
This is the path.
This is the way.

The horse blinks,
chews,
lowers their head.
Not in submission,
but in the arc of pendulation.

Learning,
true learning,
feels like this—
not forced,
but followed.
Not driven,
but drawn.

Step by step,
loop by loop,
you build a habit not of obedience
but of seeking.

And in that seeking
lies the quiet joy
of a nervous system
allowed to explore,
to choose,
to change.

This is the drift—
the neurochemical current
that shapes behavior
without breaking spirit.

And it flows both ways.

HPA Axis (Hypothalamic-Pituitary-Adrenal Axis)

The **Hypothalamic-Pituitary-Adrenal (HPA) axis** is a central component of the equine stress response system, crucial in how horses perceive, react to, and recover from stressors. As an integral part of the neuroendocrine system, the **HPA axis** orchestrates both physiological and behavioral responses to perceived threats, fears, and environmental challenges. Its primary role is to maintain homeostasis by adapting to stressors, ranging from sudden noises or isolation from herd companions to the demands encountered during training sessions. Upon detecting a stressor, the HPA axis initiates a cascade of hormonal signals, equipping the horse with the necessary energy and physiological adjustments to cope effectively.

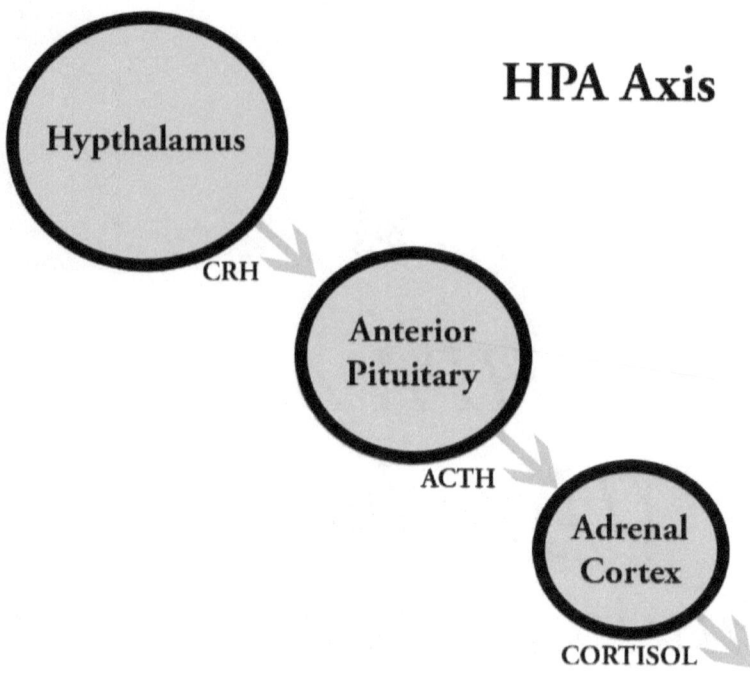

HPA Axis

At the heart of the HPA axis lies an intricate network involving three critical structures: the hypothalamus, the pituitary gland, and the adrenal glands. Stress perception begins in the hypothalamus, specifically within the **paraventricular nucleus (PVN)**, which responds by secreting **corticotropin-releasing hormone (CRH)**. This neuropeptide travels via the hypophyseal portal system to the anterior pituitary gland, triggering the release of **adrenocorticotropic hormone (ACTH)**. Subsequently, ACTH circulates through the bloodstream to the **adrenal cortex**, prompting secretion of cortisol, the primary **glucocorticoid** in horses. Cortisol's actions are extensive, facilitating energy mobilization through gluconeogenesis, modulating immune responses, and influencing cardiovascular and central nervous system function to prepare the animal for rapid and effective responses. Neurologically, cortisol interacts with limbic structures, such as the amygdala and hippocampus, influencing emotional memory formation and vigilance.

Under acute stress conditions, the rapid elevation of cortisol enhances vigilance, facilitates quick decision-making, and primes the horse for either escape or defensive behaviors essential for survival. However, sustained or chronic activation of the HPA axis due to persistent or repeated stressors—including excessive training pressures, prolonged social isolation, or suboptimal management conditions—can lead to detrimental effects. Chronic elevation of cortisol can suppress immune function, disrupt normal metabolic processes, and adversely impact cognitive functions by impairing neuroplasticity in brain regions such as the hippocampus. Consequently, prolonged stress exposure may result in maladaptive behaviors, including stereotypies, learned helplessness, aggression, hyper-reactivity, and social withdrawal. These behaviors, often misinterpreted as stubbornness or defiance in training contexts, can be indicative of underlying chronic physiological stress responses.

Incorporating knowledge of the HPA axis into evidence-based approaches emphasizes the importance of optimizing training practices and managing equine welfare by minimizing chronic stress. Effective training methods incorporate gradual habituation, clear and consistent reinforcement, and management practices aimed at reducing unnecessary stress. Recognizing behaviors related to HPA axis activation as physiological rather than deliberate acts of resistance promotes humane, informed approaches to training. Ultimately, careful management of the HPA axis enhances horses' capacity for learning and mitigates risks of stress-related pathologies.

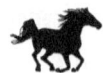

Long Term Potentiation (LTP) and Memory Formation

Learning and memory are fundamental for a horse's ability to successfully interact with its environment, adapt behaviorally, and respond effectively to training. At a cellular level, these cognitive processes are largely mediated by **long-term potentiation (LTP)**, a neurobiological phenomenon that strengthens synaptic connections between neurons through repeated and coordinated activation. LTP embodies the principle of Hebbian learning, often summarized as "Neurons that fire together, wire together," laying the neural groundwork for memory consolidation, habit formation, and skill acquisition in horses.

Primarily occurring in the hippocampus, a critical structure for spatial memory, navigation, and associative learning, LTP establishes long-lasting enhancements in synaptic strength following repeated neuronal stimulation. However, this synaptic plasticity extends beyond the hippocampus, involving regions such as the cerebellum, basal ganglia, and sensory cortices—areas responsible for motor control, habit formation, and sensory processing, respectively. For instance, when a horse repeatedly experiences a specific training cue, such as gentle pressure from a rein, the neural circuits mediating the response become increasingly efficient, allowing the horse to execute the behavior more swiftly and automatically over time.

Neurochemically, LTP is intricately linked to the dynamics of neurotransmitters and their receptors, particularly the glutamate-mediated **NMDA** and **AMPA** receptors. Early learning phases predominantly involve AMPA receptors, which rapidly respond to glutamate by allowing **sodium ions (Na^+)** to enter postsynaptic neurons, causing immediate excitatory effects and initial learning responses. As learning progresses and stimuli become repetitive and more strongly associated, NMDA receptors become critically involved. Initially blocked by **magnesium ions (Mg^{2+})** at resting membrane potentials, these receptors require substantial and repeated synaptic activation to depolarize the postsynaptic neuron enough to expel the Mg^{2+} block. Once unblocked, NMDA receptors allow **calcium ions (Ca^{2+})** into the neuron, activating intracellular signaling pathways that strengthen synaptic connections by increasing receptor density, promoting dendritic spine growth, and facilitating the creation of new synaptic contacts. These structural and functional changes form stable neural pathways necessary for long-term memory formation and behavioral conditioning.

For practical horse training, LTP signifies that consistent, repeated training interactions over time—paired with clearly defined cues and reinforcements—lead to stronger and more durable neural pathways. A young horse first introduced to halter training initially experiences novel and weakly established neural circuits associated with interpreting pressure-and-relief cues. With regular, predictable reinforcement, these pathways become robust, reducing cognitive effort and transforming the initially conscious, deliberate action into an automatic response, akin to how humans acquire motor skills through repeated practice.

Beyond synaptic changes alone, the successful formation of enduring memories in horses critically depends upon the memory consolidation process. Initially fragile and transient, short-term memories stabilize into long-term storage primarily through hippocampal replay mechanisms during periods of rest and sleep. Sleep, particularly **rapid-eye-movement (REM) sleep**, facilitates this consolidation, allowing the hippocampus to re-activate neural patterns associated with recent experiences, thereby reinforcing and stabilizing the memory traces. Hence, horses typically exhibit improved performance following rest periods, highlighting rest as a vital training component.

Neuroendocrinological factors significantly modulate LTP and memory formation, particularly the horse's emotional state and stress levels. Elevated stress, signaled through increased cortisol secretion, can inhibit synaptic plasticity, impair LTP, and compromise memory consolidation by negatively affecting hippocampal function. Conversely, emotionally rewarding experiences stimulate dopamine release, enhancing LTP by increasing neuronal excitability and synaptic efficiency. Dopamine, associated with motivation and reward anticipation, creates favorable conditions for strong memory encoding. Oxytocin, another neurohormone linked to safety and positive social interactions, further supports robust memory formation by reinforcing positive emotional contexts during training.

Therefore, trainers aiming to maximize learning efficacy must strategically balance training intensity with careful stress management, creating environments that foster positive emotional experiences and minimize cortisol release. Employing training methods grounded in neuroscientific principles, trainers ensure the horse's brain engages optimally, facilitating efficient and enduring learning.

Ultimately, comprehending the mechanisms of LTP and neuroendocrine influences empowers trainers and handlers to optimize their training methodologies. Recognizing that training fundamentally involves restructuring and strengthening neural networks emphasizes the necessity of patience, consistency, and scientifically informed approaches. Through careful application of these principles, horses develop the neural frameworks necessary for reliably performing trained behaviors, demonstrating that successful training transcends behavioral modifications and fundamentally reshapes neural architecture. More than reshaping behavior, you are reshaping the brain itself.

SECTION II
Sensory Processing, Emotion, and Behavior

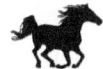

Sensory Perception and Processing

"A new paradigm in horsemanship begins when we stop imposing our assumptions and start seeing through the horse's eyes."

—Dr. Stephen Peters

Our Separate Sensory Worlds

You and your horse live in separate worlds. Where we tend to get into trouble, is when we think that the horse is operating with a human brain and perceives the world as we do. This makes sense because the only model most of us have for comparison is our own brain. However, we cannot experience the world as the horse perceives it. We have two very different realities. Perception is defined by our senses. Thus, having different senses, horses perceive the world differently. Often, the horse is simply doing perfectly what their nervous system was designed to do. It is the human who labels the behavior with negative or positive terms. The better one understands the nervous systems underpinnings of their horse's behavior, the more one can set-up situations to optimize communication and direct behavior in a positive way for the horse and its rider. One of the keys to gaining insight into our horse's world as they experience it, is to understand what they use their senses for.

Horses experience the world through a rich tapestry of sensory information, shaped by their evolutionary history as prey animals. Their perception is finely tuned to detect environmental changes, identify potential threats, and facilitate social interactions. Each sensory modality, sight, sound, smell, touch, and proprioception, contributes to their ability to navigate their surroundings, communicate with other horses, and respond to training. Understanding the horse's sensory systems provides insight into their behavior, learning processes, and welfare needs.

Sensory receptors constantly process stimuli, which the brain organizes and interprets into perception.

Equine Vision: A Different Way of Seeing the World

Vision is among a horse's most critical senses, finely honed for survival in expansive environments where detecting subtle movements early can be lifesaving. Unlike humans, whose forward-facing eyes grant detailed but relatively limited frontal vision, horses possess large eyes positioned laterally, giving them an expansive, nearly 340-degree panoramic view. This broad visual scope enables horses to survey their surroundings with minimal head movement, a significant evolutionary advantage. However, the trade-off for such extensive peripheral vision includes two notable blind spots—one directly in front of the horse's muzzle and another immediately behind its tail—necessitating intentional head movements to monitor these zones effectively.

Horses primarily utilize monocular vision, meaning each eye independently observes a separate wide-angle view. This arrangement

SENSORY PROCESSING, EMOTION, AND BEHAVIOR

greatly enhances their ability to detect potential threats from multiple directions simultaneously but compromises their depth perception. When precise depth perception is required, horses switch to binocular vision, focusing both eyes forward to overlap their visual fields. This binocular overlap is limited, explaining why horses typically lower their heads when navigating uneven ground or stepping onto unfamiliar surfaces, such as trailer ramps, to better gauge depth and distance.

A distinctive characteristic of equine vision is the horizontally elongated pupil, commonly called the visual streak. This specialized adaptation significantly enhances their ability to perceive horizontal movement across vast landscapes, particularly beneficial while grazing. In contrast to humans, whose circular pupils and robust ciliary muscles allow rapid shifts in focal distance, horses have weaker ciliary muscles, restricting their ability to quickly adjust focus between near and distant objects. Consequently, horses rely heavily on head movements and specific head positioning to bring objects into clearer focus. They often tilt or cock their heads to align objects of interest with the retinal region richest in ganglion cells, analogous to how humans fix their gaze straight ahead for detailed visual inspection.

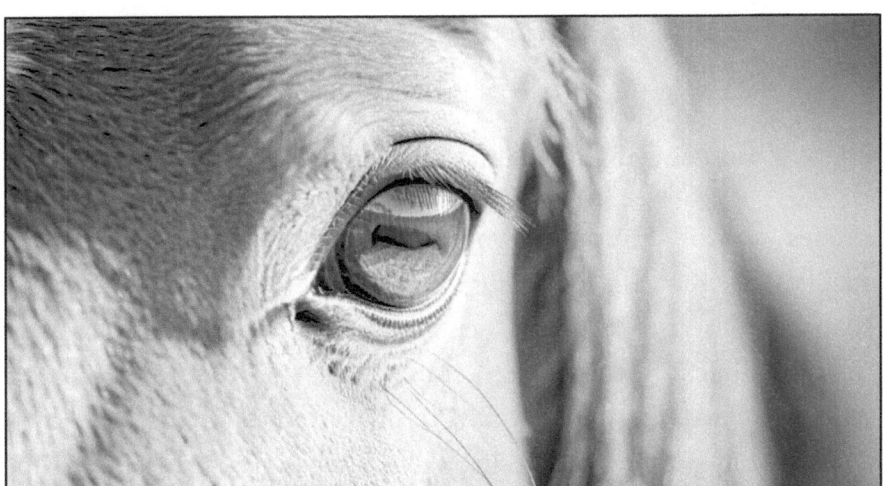

Color Perception and Visual Acuity

Horses are **dichromatic**, meaning they perceive a limited spectrum of colors. While humans have three types of cone cells (**trichromatic**) that detect red, green, and blue, horses lack the red-sensitive cones. As a result, their world consists of shades of blue and yellow, while reds and greens appear as variations of gray. This has practical implications in training and competition, where certain colored obstacles may not stand out as vividly to a horse as they do to a human. White and yellow objects tend to appear more starkly contrasted, which is why some horses may react more strongly to them.

While horses do not see the world with the same sharpness as humans, they are highly attuned to movement. Their vision has been estimated at 20/35 compared to a human with 20/20 vision, meaning their world appears slightly blurrier. This is due to the different ratio of photoreceptors in their retina; horses have a much higher proportion of rod cells to cone cells, sometimes estimated at 20:1. Rod cells specialize in detecting motion and light levels, while cone cells provide clarity and color perception. As a result, horses excel at detecting movement, particularly in low-light conditions, but their ability to discern fine details is less refined.

Night Vision and Light Adaptation

Horses possess exceptional night vision, a critical evolutionary adaptation enhancing their survival as prey animals. Central to this adaptation is the tapetum lucidum, a specialized reflective layer situated directly behind the retina. This structure functions by reflecting incoming light back through the photoreceptor cells, effectively amplifying the available light and significantly improving visual sensitivity in low-light conditions. Neurologically, this adaptation maximizes the stimulation of rod photoreceptors, the retinal cells specialized for dim-light detection, thereby allowing horses to navigate and detect potential threats effectively at night. The tapetum lucidum is also responsible for the distinctive eye shine observed when a horse's eyes reflect light in darkness.

However, this heightened night vision has a distinct neurological tradeoff. Horses experience slower pupillary reflexes and neural adaptation to sudden changes in ambient brightness compared to humans. While human visual adaptation occurs rapidly—often within mere seconds—equine visual processing, governed by their neural circuitry, requires a prolonged period, sometimes up to 30 minutes, to fully adjust from dark environments to bright conditions. This delay is primarily due to the slower neural adjustments within the retinal circuitry and visual pathways, which must recalibrate sensitivity and integration to varying illumination levels. Consequently, horses often exhibit superior visual acuity in diffuse or overcast lighting rather than intense, direct sunlight.

Complementing this adaptation is the presence of specialized anatomical features known as corpora nigra, or granula iridica. These pigmented, dark-brown or black structures, located predominantly along the dorsal margin and occasionally on the ventral edge of the iris, serve as natural filters regulating light influx. Composed of pigmented epithelial tissue, the corpora nigra protrude into the pupil to shield the retina by absorbing excessive incoming light, thereby reducing glare and enhancing visual contrast. From a neurological standpoint, this structural adaptation optimizes visual clarity by preventing overstimulation of retinal photoreceptors and the subsequent neural fatigue associated with bright, intense illumination. This feature is particularly advantageous for horses, enabling them to maintain sharp vision and heightened alertness across diverse lighting conditions encountered in their environment.

Occasionally, corpora nigra can develop fluid-filled cysts, potentially obstructing the pupil and impairing vision. Such anomalies disrupt normal visual processing and neural signaling, necessitating veterinary intervention, commonly through laser ablation, to restore unobstructed visual function.

Neural Pathways and Visual Processing

The neural wiring of equine vision further distinguishes their perception from that of humans. Visual information from each eye is transmitted to the opposite side of the brain via the **optic chiasm**, an X-shaped structure beneath the brain where the optic nerves cross. While humans also experience this crossover, a larger percentage of visual information in horses is sent **contralaterally** (to the opposite hemisphere), rather than being processed equally in both hemispheres.

Impact of Environment on Vision

Equine cranial anatomy, characterized by an elongated skull structure and laterally positioned eyes, enables horses to achieve a nearly complete panoramic field of view, particularly beneficial for continuous vigilance against predators while grazing. Neuroscientifically, consistent exposure to expansive horizons engages neural mechanisms that support optimal visual acuity at distance. In contrast, horses maintained in confined environments like stalls or barns can experience visual impoverishment, leading to neuroplastic adaptations that favor near-field vision. Prolonged absence of distant focal stimuli can prompt functional shifts within neural circuits in the visual cortex, resulting in increased prevalence of myopia (nearsightedness). The infrequency of myopia among wild or free-ranging equines underscores the neurophysiological benefits of environments that afford varied visual stimuli, reinforcing the recommendation that domesticated horses receive regular access to open spaces.

Implications for Handling and Training

An informed understanding of equine visual neurobiology has significant implications for optimizing horse-human interactions, refining training methodologies, and enhancing safety protocols. Horses process visual stimuli in a manner distinctively different from humans; specifically, their heightened sensitivity to peripheral motion relies heavily on magnocellular visual pathways specialized for detecting rapid movement, rather than the parvocellular pathways that humans utilize for color perception and fine detail discernment. As a result, equine startle responses are commonly triggered by sudden or unexpected peripheral movement rather than detailed static imagery.

Handlers and trainers must thoughtfully account for horses' panoramic visual field, anatomical blind spots—such as immediately in front of their face and directly behind their body—and limited depth perception, particularly at close range. By consciously approaching horses within their visual field, allowing sufficient time for recognition, and methodically introducing novel stimuli bilaterally, trainers support the equine brain's ability to encode, habituate, and consolidate visual experiences effectively. This approach leverages a nuanced appreciation of the neural underpinnings of equine visual perception, making for safer and more productive interactions.

Hearing – Auditory Perception in Horses

A horse's auditory system is a finely tuned sensory apparatus, critical for survival, communication, and interaction with its environment. As prey animals, horses have evolved to rely heavily on their acute hearing to detect potential threats before they come into view. Their highly mobile pinnae, which can rotate independently in a nearly 180-degree arc, serve as biological radar dishes, funneling sound waves toward the inner ear. With at least ten muscles dedicated to each ear's movement, horses can rapidly shift their auditory attention from one source to another, allowing them to monitor multiple sound cues simultaneously.

One of the defining characteristics of equine hearing is its sensitivity to high-frequency sounds. Horses detect a wider range of frequencies than humans, with an upper hearing limit of approximately 33 kHz, compared to a human's 20 kHz. This ability enables them to perceive subtle environmental cues, such as the ultrasonic sounds of insects or the faint rustle of dry leaves and snapping twigs underfoot, noises that could indicate the presence of a predator. Their auditory acuity allows them to react swiftly, often stopping mid-motion, lifting their heads, and directing their ears toward the source of a sound. While humans may rely more on visual confirmation, horses instinctively trust their auditory system to assess potential danger before engaging their other senses.

Horses utilize **binaural hearing**, meaning that their brains process input from both ears simultaneously to determine the direction and distance of a sound source. By comparing the slight differences in

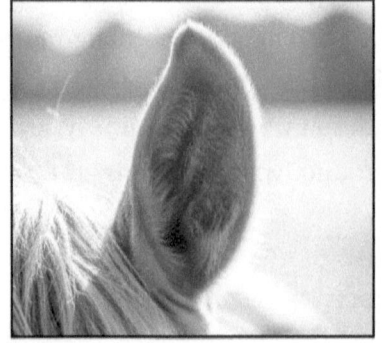

timing and intensity of a sound as it reaches each ear, horses form a spatial map of their surroundings. However, despite this ability, research suggests that horses are not as precise as humans when it comes to sound localization. While they can detect the general direction of a noise, they may struggle to pinpoint its exact origin with the same accuracy that humans achieve through our stationary ears.

There is also growing speculation that horses may perceive certain low-frequency vibrations through their hooves rather than through conventional auditory pathways. This would be akin to a form of **proprioceptive sound perception**, similar to how elephants detect seismic activity through the ground. The ability to feel the distant rumble of approaching hooves or an oncoming storm may play a role in a horse's rapid responses to environmental changes, even when there is no obvious auditory cue to the human observer.

Auditory perception in horses is not solely limited to threat detection; it also plays a fundamental role in communication. Horses are highly responsive to vocal cues, both from conspecifics and humans. Studies indicate that horses can recognize individual voices, differentiating between familiar and unfamiliar vocal patterns. Additionally, horses integrate auditory and visual cues when identifying human handlers, a skill that reflects their capacity for cross-modal perception. This means that a horse does not rely on just one sense but rather combines auditory information with visual recognition to form a more complete understanding of its surroundings.

Hearing loss, although less frequently studied in equines compared to other species, is an area of increasing interest in equine welfare. Certain coat patterns, particularly those linked to the **splashed white and frame overo genes** in American Paint Horses, have been associated with congenital deafness. Additionally, while age-related hearing loss has been well-documented in other mammals, it remains an underexplored topic in horses, with anecdotal reports suggesting that some older horses may develop diminished auditory sensitivity.

Environmental noise pollution, often overlooked in equine management, can also impact horses' auditory experience. Wind turbines, ultrasonic pest deterrents, and even certain types of vehicle noise generate high-frequency sounds that fall outside of human hearing but may be well within the auditory range of horses. Exposure to such persistent, unnatural noises could contribute to stress or sensory fatigue in equines, especially in confined settings where escape from the auditory stimulus is not possible.

Olfaction in Horses

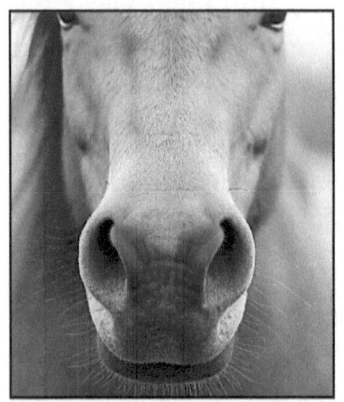

Olfaction, or the sense of smell, is a vital sensory modality for horses, underpinning their social interactions, environmental awareness, and survival instincts. The equine olfactory system is highly developed, enabling horses to process complex chemical signals that inform their behavior and decision-making. From identifying conspecifics to assessing potential threats in their surroundings, the horse's acute sense of smell plays a fundamental role in daily life.

Horses possess an extensive olfactory epithelium, a specialized tissue in the nasal cavity responsible for detecting airborne molecules. This structure allows them to perceive and interpret a diverse array of scents with remarkable sensitivity. A critical component of their olfactory apparatus is the **vomeronasal organ (VNO)**, also known as Jacobson's organ. This auxiliary chemoreceptor system is dedicated to detecting pheromones, chemical signals that convey social and reproductive information. Activation of the VNO often manifests in the Flehmen response, a characteristic behavior where a horse curls its upper lip and inhales, facilitating deeper scent analysis. This response is particularly common in stallions assessing the reproductive status of mares, but it is also observed in other social and exploratory contexts.

Olfactory information in mammals, including horses and humans, is initially processed in an ipsilateral fashion. This means that sensory input from the right nostril is received and processed by the right olfactory bulb and input from the left nostril by the left bulb. Unlike most other sensory systems, olfaction does not cross over to the contralateral side at the level of the brainstem or thalamus. Instead, the primary olfactory projections—those from the olfactory bulb to the olfactory cortex—remain on the same side of the brain. However, as olfactory information progresses to higher-order processing centers, such as the piriform cortex and entorhinal cortex, it is shared between the two hemispheres via the anterior commissure. This interhemispheric connection allows for bilateral integration of olfactory information, supporting a unified perception of odor despite the initially ipsilateral processing pathway.

Social interactions among horses are strongly influenced by olfactory cues. Research indicates that horses can recognize individuals based on scent, allowing them to differentiate between familiar and unfamiliar herd members. This capability extends to fecal and urine marking, wherein horses may show a stronger reaction to the scent of dominant or aggressive conspecifics. Such scent-based recognition mechanisms are critical in establishing and maintaining social hierarchies within herds.

Beyond social communication, the equine olfactory system plays a crucial role in environmental perception. Horses can detect changes in their surroundings through scent cues, alerting them to potential dangers such as predators. Studies have demonstrated that horses exhibit heightened vigilance when exposed to the scent of natural predators, such as wolf urine. This innate response underscores the evolutionary significance of olfaction in equine survival, allowing horses to anticipate and react to threats even in the absence of direct visual or auditory confirmation.

In addition to processing equine and environmental odors, horses are also sensitive to human scent. Emerging research suggests that horses can detect and respond to human emotional states through olfactory cues. For example, stress-related compounds present in human sweat may elicit behavioral changes in horses, influencing their responses during handling and training. This finding highlights the importance of emotional regulation and composure in horse-human interactions, as a handler's physiological state may inadvertently impact a horse's behavior and perception of safety.

Furthermore, olfaction plays a role in horses' ability to locate water sources, identify palatable food, and avoid toxic substances. While vision and taste contribute to dietary choices, scent perception helps horses discriminate between safe and potentially harmful plants. This function is particularly relevant in free-ranging or feral populations, where horses must rely on their sensory faculties to navigate diverse landscapes and forage effectively.

The olfactory capabilities of horses, though less studied than their visual or auditory systems, represent an essential aspect of their sensory world. From reinforcing social bonds to detecting threats and influencing human-equine relationships, olfaction serves as a fundamental mechanism for communication and survival.

Vibrissae

The hair on our head and the whiskers on our face are pelagic hair, the equivalent of fur or wool. What horses also have that we don't are Vibrissae, which is Latin for "to vibrate".

Vibrissae are specialized sensory hairs found around a horse's muzzle, including the upper and lower lips, nostrils, and around the eyes. Unlike ordinary body hairs, vibrissae are deeply embedded in the skin and connected to a dense network of nerves, making them highly sensitive tactile structures. Each whisker is rooted in a specialized follicle rich in blood vessels and sensory nerves, forming what is known as a sinus hair follicle. These whiskers are much thicker and longer than regular hairs and have direct connections to the trigeminal nerve (cranial nerve V), which transmits tactile information to the brain. The muzzle, particularly around the lips and nostrils, has an extremely high concentration of vibrissae, allowing horses to navigate their environment and detect objects in close proximity, even in low-light conditions.

The primary function of vibrissae is to aid in environmental exploration, as horses use their whiskers to sense objects in their immediate surroundings, particularly when grazing, drinking, or interacting with other horses. This is crucial because horses have limited binocular vision and a blind spot directly in front of their muzzle, making tactile cues an important source of information. Vibrissae also play a key role in foraging and food selection, helping horses detect and discriminate textures, which enables 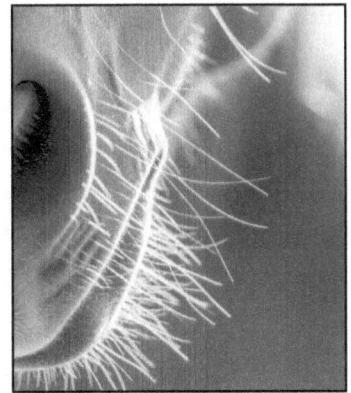 them to distinguish between edible and non-edible items. They are particularly useful for locating small food particles, ensuring efficient grazing and feeding. Additionally, vibrissae enhance social and grooming behaviors, as horses often use their muzzle and whiskers to investigate and interact with other horses, particularly during mutual grooming. These whiskers improve their ability to detect subtle changes in pressure, movement, or texture on another horse's body. The supraorbital vibrissae, located above the eyes, act as early warning systems to prevent eye injuries by detecting approaching objects before contact occurs. Contact with vibrissae can trigger avoidance reflexes, helping horses prevent injuries from foreign objects or potential threats.

Exploration of Novel Objects

When encountering a novel object, a horse engages in a systematic process of sensory exploration, primarily relying on olfaction and tactile feedback to assess its properties. Initially, the horse will use its highly developed sense of smell, powered by its large olfactory bulb and Jacobson's organ (vomeronasal organ), to detect any chemical traces that might indicate whether the object has been handled, carries a familiar scent, or has any biological relevance, such as plant material. Following this, the horse will contact its vibrissae—specialized sensory hairs on the muzzle—allowing it to detect subtle variations in texture and shape with remarkable sensitivity. Next, the upper lip, which has a high density of **mechanoreceptors**, is used to manipulate and further explore the object. The lip's fine motor control enables delicate interactions, much like a human's fingertips. Finally, the horse may gently take the object between its teeth, applying pressure to assess its density, weight, and overall composition. This investigative sequence mirrors the way humans rely on their hands to explore new objects, integrating multiple sensory inputs to form a comprehensive understanding. This process is essential for curiosity-driven learning, helping the horse determine whether an unfamiliar object is safe, stable, or potentially hazardous.

Horses also rely on these highly sensitive mechanoreceptors in their lips to differentiate between edible plant material and inedible substances such as dirt and rocks. These specialized sensory receptors, particularly Merkel cells and Meissner corpuscles, provide detailed tactile feedback, allowing the horse to assess texture, density, and pliability with remarkable precision. As they graze, horses use their mobile and prehensile upper lip to explore and sift through vegetation, detecting subtle differences in resistance and structure. When encountering plant material, the mechanoreceptors signal the presence of pliable, fibrous textures indicative of grass, leaves, or stems, triggering further investigation with their incisors. In contrast, when they encounter hard, unyielding surfaces such as rocks or compacted soil, the sensory input helps them reject these objects before ingestion. This finely tuned sensory system reduces the risk of accidentally consuming harmful debris and enhances foraging efficiency, ensuring that horses select nutrient-rich food sources while minimizing potential digestive complications.

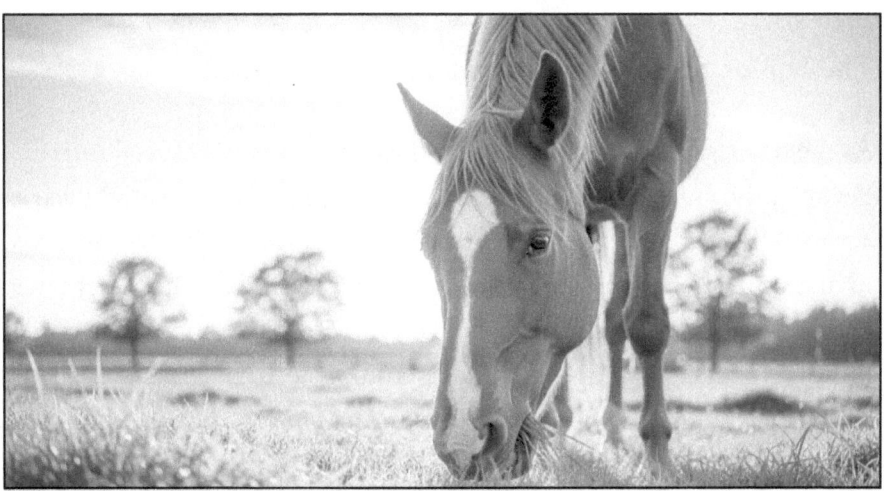

Despite their functional significance, vibrissae have often been trimmed or removed in some equestrian disciplines for aesthetic purposes, a practice that has become increasingly controversial. Scientific evidence suggests that removing vibrissae impairs a horse's ability to navigate and detect objects, increasing the risk of facial trauma, difficulty in feeding, and overall sensory deprivation. In response to these concerns, the International Equestrian Federation (FEI) banned the trimming of horse whiskers in 2021, citing welfare implications. Several European countries, including Germany, France, and Switzerland, have also prohibited vibrissae removal under animal welfare laws. Given their critical function in tactile sensation, foraging, social interactions, and self-protection, trimming or removing whiskers is now widely regarded as a welfare concern.

The sensory neurons associated with vibrissae require consistent stimulation to maintain function, and their prolonged absence may result in atrophy or failure to integrate fully into the horse's somatosensory system. Since the developing nervous system is highly plastic, early removal can disrupt normal sensory mapping in the brain, leading to a permanent reduction in tactile acuity.

The Equine Sensory System and Tactile Perception

As the horse's largest sensory organ, the skin serves as a crucial interface between the animal and its environment. Equine skin sensitivity varies across different body regions, with heightened responsiveness observed in areas such as the muzzle, withers, and lower limbs. This heightened tactile perception influences social interactions, learning, and training responsiveness, making an understanding of the horse's sensory experience integral to optimizing welfare and performance.

The Equine Somatosensory System: Understanding Touch in Reinforcement

Horses possess an exceptionally refined somatosensory system, with their skin containing a dense network of mechanoreceptors that detect touch, pressure, vibration, and pain. This tactile sensitivity plays a fundamental role in equine communication, social bonding, and learning. One of the most powerful forms of positive reinforcement for horses is physical touch in the form of rubbing and scratching. These actions stimulate the release of oxytocin, the neuropeptide associated with safety, trust, and social bonding, as well as serotonin, which contributes to emotional balance and relaxation.

The neurobiological effects of rubbing and scratching are rooted in natural equine behaviors. Mutual grooming (allogrooming) among horses is a critical component of herd dynamics, strengthening social bonds and reducing stress. The repetitive scratching motion mimics the sensations horses experience when engaging in allogrooming with a trusted companion. Additionally, foals experience tactile reinforcement from their mothers, particularly through licking, which provides not only comfort but also a strong social attachment. These natural interactions have direct neurochemical benefits, reinforcing positive emotional states and deepening relationships.

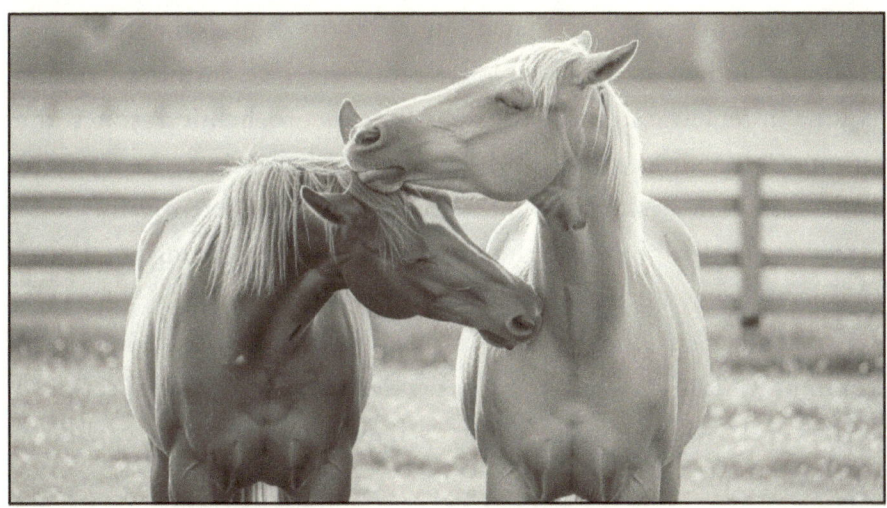

Conversely, slapping and patting—common human behaviors meant to express praise—lack any natural analogue in equine interactions. Unlike rubbing or grooming, abrupt tapping or slapping can trigger an involuntary startle response, leading to a spike in norepinephrine, the neurotransmitter associated with arousal and vigilance. Rather than experiencing this as a reward, many horses find these actions aversive, leading to a learned tolerance rather than genuine positive reinforcement. Over time, horses may habituate to patting, appearing indifferent or accepting, but this is not the same as finding it rewarding. Instead of promoting relaxation and trust, such actions may subtly contribute to tension, confusion, or even conditioned suppression of responses. Licking and chewing after being patted or slapped can mistakenly be interpreted as a sign of positive reinforcement, believing the horse is relaxed and appreciative. However, in many cases, the horse licks and chews because the patting has become a signal that the excessive control, spurring, yanking, or dominance has ceased. This response is not an indication of pleasure but rather a shift from heightened sympathetic arousal back toward a state of relief and recovery.

By understanding how the equine somatosensory system is wired to respond to different forms of touch, handlers can use reinforcement strategies that align with the horse's neurobiology. Rubbing and scratching not only replicate the comfort of natural equine interactions but also encourage neurochemical states that promote learning, trust, and emotional well-being. In contrast, behaviors such as slapping and patting may inadvertently introduce stress signals, emphasizing the importance of recognizing the horse's perspective when using touch as reinforcement.

Tactile perception also plays a crucial role in training and communication between horse and rider. The precise application of tactile cues, whether from a rider's hands, legs, or seat, can direct movement and refine responses. Understanding the horse's sensitivity to touch allows trainers to use subtle aids and minimal well-defined cues rather than excessive pressure, thereby improving communication and responsiveness.

Mechanoreceptors and Their Function in Tactile Sensitivity

Horses possess a highly sophisticated network of **mechanoreceptors**, enabling exceptional sensitivity and rapid responsiveness to tactile stimuli ranging from subtle touches to deeper pressure and vibrations. Four primary mechanoreceptor types underpin this acute tactile awareness. **Merkel's disks** detect gentle touch and sustained pressure, allowing horses precise tactile discrimination crucial for assessing their environment. **Meissner's corpuscles** respond to subtle touch and lower-frequency vibrations, facilitating the detection of dynamic environmental changes. **Ruffini's corpuscles** sense warmth and skin stretch, contributing significantly to proprioceptive feedback, essential for coordinated movement and spatial awareness. **Pacinian corpuscles**, specialized for recognizing rapid vibrations and sudden deep pressure, initiate swift reflexive responses, crucial for predator evasion.

These mechanoreceptors primarily communicate through large, heavily myelinated axons, ensuring rapid signal transmission to the central nervous system (CNS) and enabling immediate behavioral responses. However, some mechanoreceptors utilize slower-conducting unmyelinated fibers, resulting in prolonged, sustained sensory perception. This dual speed signaling ensures horses remain continuously attuned to their surroundings, a vital adaptation given their evolutionary status as prey animals requiring constant vigilance.

Aversive Tactile Stimuli and Welfare Considerations

Positive tactile experiences significantly enhance horse welfare, yet aversive tactile stimuli can negatively impact horses' psychological and physical states. Excessive or inappropriate tactile inputs, such as tightly fitted restrictive nosebands, harsh bits, and whip usage, have been shown to elicit pain, stress, and behavioral responses indicative of distress, including tail swishing, head tossing, and resistance behaviors. The perception of pain varies considerably between individual horses due to genetic predisposition, prior experiences, health conditions, and environmental factors. **Nociceptors**, the specialized sensory neurons responsible for detecting noxious stimuli, fall into four primary categories: mechanical nociceptors sensitive to intense pressure, thermal nociceptors responding to extreme temperature variations, chemical nociceptors triggered by inflammatory substances and irritants, and polymodal nociceptors, capable of responding to multiple forms of painful stimuli.

Repeated exposure to aversive or painful stimuli can induce neural sensitization, enhancing pain perception and exacerbating stress responses through neuroplastic changes within the sensory pathways. Conversely, strategically applied desensitization techniques facilitate neural habituation, diminishing exaggerated responses to non-threatening stimuli, thereby fostering resilience and adaptability in horses.

Neuroendocrine Influence on Sensory Perception

The neuroendocrine system significantly influences equine sensory perception and behavioral responses. Hormonal variations, particularly the release of stress-related hormones such as cortisol and norepinephrine, heighten sensory sensitivity by lowering detection thresholds. This heightened vigilance facilitates rapid responses to potential threats, enhancing survival capabilities in challenging environments. Conversely, environments that foster calmness and security promote optimal neuroendocrine conditions, facilitating neural states conducive to effective learning, memory consolidation, and overall welfare. Incorporating awareness of these neuroendocrine mechanisms into training practices ensures horses remain engaged, receptive, and emotionally balanced, optimizing their learning potential and reducing unnecessary stress.

Proprioception: Awareness of Movement and Balance

Proprioception, the intrinsic sense of body position and movement, is integral to equine coordination, balance, and athletic performance. Specialized proprioceptive receptors within muscles (**muscle spindles**), tendons (**Golgi tendon organs**), and joint capsules continuously relay critical positional information to the CNS, informing precise motor control and adjustments. The vestibular system within the inner ear complements this proprioceptive information by providing essential feedback regarding balance, equilibrium, and spatial orientation. Robust proprioceptive capabilities enable horses to modulate stride length, adeptly navigate varied terrains, and rapidly recover balance following unexpected disturbances. Training methodologies designed to enhance proprioceptive acuity—such as groundwork, obstacle navigation, and exposure to varied topography and footing surfaces—can significantly bolster coordination, proprioceptive awareness, and injury resilience.

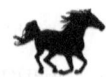

Safety First: The Neurobiology of Fear, Stress, and Emotional Well-being in Horses

"A Horse Remembers"
by Dr. Stephen Peters

She stood alone at the far end of the paddock—still, frozen, somewhere else.
The same spot she returned to every day.

To most, it looked like a simple habit.
But to me... it was a footprint etched into the nervous system.

You see, a horse doesn't remember the way we do.
There are no words. No timeline. No story.

There is only Sensation. Emotion. Pattern.
And when a moment is flooded with cortisol, fear, and uncertainty,
the memory is etched deep by the amygdala.

Especially after being *"taught a lesson"* more than once.

She wasn't just standing there—
she was checked out, numbed out…
not living in the now,
but trapped in the past.

But there is hope.
With patience, softness, and the right approach—
through safety, consistency, and time—
that memory can be reshaped.

Not erased. Not forgotten.
But softened, reframed, and rewired.

That is the quiet power of working with the brain and nervous system.
Not command, but connection.
Not force, but understanding.

And sometimes, it begins…
by simply standing still.

Safety is the cornerstone of equine welfare. The intricate interplay of neurobiology and neuroendocrinology dictates how horses perceive, respond to, and recover from stress and fear. As prey animals, horses rely on a finely tuned nervous system that balances vigilance with relaxation. Their ability to feel safe in their environment profoundly impacts their behavior, learning, and overall well-being. This chapter explores the mechanisms that govern fear and stress, including learned helplessness, Polyvagal Theory, trigger stacking, the cardiac nervous system, the window of tolerance, the Yerkes-Dodson Law, orienting responses, trauma, and conditioned fear responses, and emphasizes the critical role of safety in fostering emotional regulation and resilience.

Emotional Regulation and Homeostasis in the Horse

The foundation of emotional regulation, learning, and resilience in horses is built upon their perception of safety. Ensuring that a horse feels secure in its environment not only prevents chronic stress but also enhances their ability to form positive social bonds, engage in effective training, and maintain physical health. The neuroendocrine system plays a pivotal role in these processes, as hormones such as cortisol, oxytocin, and vasopressin influence a horse's ability to manage fear, stress, and social connection. However, horses can also become victims of their own neurochemistry, with prolonged stress causing them to revert to default survival states. By fostering environments that support autonomic balance, recognizing signs of dysregulation, and implementing ethical training practices, we can create safer, more trusting relationships with horses. This approach enhances not only their resilience but also their ability to engage, learn, and thrive in human care.

Horses, like all living organisms, rely on the fundamental biological principle of homeostasis to maintain stability within their internal environment. Homeostasis is the process by which physiological systems regulate themselves to ensure optimal function despite external and internal challenges. This delicate balance is managed by an intricate interplay of the nervous, endocrine, and immune systems, all working in concert to maintain stability in core bodily functions such as temperature regulation, hydration, energy balance, and stress response. Without effective self-regulation, a horse's ability to perform, recover, and remain in good health would be significantly compromised.

A key factor in maintaining homeostasis is the horse's perception of safety. A sense of security allows the nervous system to remain balanced, preventing excessive stress responses. When a horse feels safe, the parasympathetic nervous system can function optimally, enabling relaxation, digestion, and recovery. Conversely, when a horse experiences chronic stress due to uncertainty, isolation, or improper handling, the sympathetic nervous system remains activated, leading to long-term health and behavioral issues.

The hypothalamic-pituitary-adrenal (HPA) axis plays a fundamental role in the endocrine regulation of stress responses. When a horse perceives a threat, the hypothalamus signals the pituitary gland to release adrenocorticotropic hormone (ACTH), which in turn stimulates the adrenal glands to produce cortisol. Cortisol serves essential functions, including mobilizing energy reserves and modulating immune responses. However, chronic elevation of cortisol due to sustained stress can lead to immune suppression, metabolic disorders, muscle wastage, and increased fear responses, making stress management critical for equine welfare.

When horses encounter novel objects, especially those that are not readily identifiable or that exhibit movement, these stimuli are immediately prioritized by the Reticular Activating System (RAS). This system acts as a critical filter for sensory input, ensuring that potential threats or unfamiliar stimuli receive heightened attention. Understanding this neural prioritization can help us design training and handling strategies that minimize stress while fostering curiosity and trust.

Additionally, activation of the lateral hypothalamus contributes to sympathetic arousal by stimulating norepinephrine-producing neurons in the locus coeruleus. This cascade enhances vigilance, heightening awareness and readiness to respond to potential threats.

Horses can also become victims of their own neurochemistry, particularly when stress hormones dominate their physiological and behavioral responses. If a horse is repeatedly exposed to stressful conditions, its neuroendocrine system may become dysregulated, leading to an exaggerated or prolonged stress response. Sympathetic arousal causes the secretion of glucocorticoids as a response to stress. The sympathetic stress response can get stuck in the "on" position resulting in chronic stress This can manifest as hyperreactivity, excessive vigilance, or an inability to recover from stressful encounters, making the horse more prone to reverting to default survival states such as fight, flight, or freeze. This automatic response, dictated by neurochemical shifts, highlights the importance of ensuring that horses feel safe in their environment to prevent maladaptive patterns from developing.

Dopamine and Fear Extinction

Recent advances in neuroscience have unveiled dopamine's critical and previously underappreciated role in fear extinction, significantly reshaping our understanding of how horses overcome anxiety and learn from experiences. Traditionally viewed primarily through its functions in reward-seeking behavior and motivation, dopamine is now recognized as pivotal in shaping emotional memories—specifically, in the process of extinguishing fearful responses. Researchers have identified that the ventral tegmental area (VTA), a central hub of dopamine production, directly engages specific neuronal populations within the amygdala, facilitating the extinction of fear memories. This intricate circuitry underscores that reward pathways and emotional learning systems are deeply intertwined.

In practical terms, when a horse experiences fear—whether from previous trauma, negative training experiences, or stressful environments—its brain encodes these experiences within neural circuits, making future fear responses more likely. Dopamine, when activated appropriately through carefully structured reward-based training, helps the horse's brain dissociate fear-inducing stimuli from negative outcomes. Each successful exposure paired with positive reinforcement not only provides immediate relief but actively remodels neural pathways within the amygdala, progressively diminishing fear responses over time. This neuroplastic process of fear extinction via dopamine-driven pathways is foundational in humane, effective training methods.

The implications of this neuroscience are profound for trainers and horse owners alike. Conventional approaches that rely heavily on punishment or overly stressful methods can inadvertently reinforce fear memories by creating persistent stress responses, diminishing dopamine's efficacy in fear extinction processes. Conversely, thoughtfully integrated reward-based strategies that consistently trigger dopaminergic pathways enable horses to experience safer emotional landscapes. These methods encourage exploratory behaviors, curiosity, and confidence—qualities rooted in healthy dopamine dynamics. Consequently, horses become better equipped emotionally and neurologically to handle future stressors.

Learned helplessness is a psychological phenomenon in which an individual, after repeated exposure to uncontrollable and aversive stimuli, develops a passive resignation to their circumstances, ceasing to attempt escape or exert control even when opportunities arise. This concept was first identified by psychologists Martin Seligman and Steven Maier in the 1960s through experiments involving dogs exposed to inescapable shocks. Initially, the dogs attempted to escape, but after repeated failure, they stopped trying altogether, even when later given the opportunity to avoid the shocks. This response, characterized by a loss of motivation and an expectation that efforts will not change the outcome, has since been recognized in a variety of contexts, including human psychology, education, and animal welfare.

A key factor in learned helplessness is the role of **locus of control**, a psychological concept that refers to an individual's belief about the degree to which they have control over their environment and life events. **An internal locus of control** is the belief that one's actions directly influence outcomes, leading to a sense of autonomy, motivation, and resilience. In contrast, **an external locus of control** is the perception that outcomes are dictated by external forces such as fate, luck, or the actions of others, fostering passivity and reduced motivation. Learned helplessness occurs when an individual, whether human or animal, shifts from an internal locus of control to an external one, believing that no amount of effort will change their circumstances.

In humans, learned helplessness is closely linked to mental health conditions such as depression and anxiety disorders, where individuals may feel powerless to alter their situations. Those with a strong internal locus of control tend to be more proactive and resilient in the face of challenges, while those with an external locus of control may be more prone to feelings of helplessness and despair. Research has demonstrated that restoring a sense of control, even in small ways, can mitigate the effects of learned helplessness, underscoring the critical role of agency in psychological well-being.

In the realm of animal behavior, learned helplessness is of particular concern in equine welfare and training. Horses, as prey animals, rely on their flight response to avoid threats and discomfort. However, when subjected to training methods that involve excessive punishment, persistent restraint, or inescapable pressure, they may enter a state of learned helplessness. This condition is often mistaken for compliance, as the horse may appear calm, obedient, or even "well-trained;" rather, it has ceased attempting to engage with its environment due to past experiences of futility.

For example, a horse that has been repeatedly subjected to harsh use of bits, relentless use of spurs, or excessive whipping may initially resist, attempt to flee, or display signs of distress. However, if these efforts are consistently ignored or punished, the horse may eventually stop reacting altogether. Instead of resisting, the animal may stand motionless, lower its head, or exhibit a dull expression, behaviors that can be easily misinterpreted as signs of submission rather than indicators of psychological suppression. This learned passivity is not a sign of trust or respect but rather a manifestation of stress and resignation, highlighting the ethical concerns surrounding coercive training practices.

The transition from an internal to an external locus of control in horses is particularly damaging because it disrupts their ability to engage in natural problem-solving behaviors and erodes their sense of agency. A horse with an internal locus of control is more likely to explore its environment, respond to training with curiosity, and learn effectively. Conversely, a horse that has been conditioned into an external locus of control through aversive experiences may no longer attempt to influence its surroundings, leading to a dull, robotic demeanor. This shift not only affects their emotional state but also their ability to learn, as a horse that no longer believes its actions matter is less likely to respond to cues or engage with training in a meaningful way.

The long-term consequences of learned helplessness in horses are significant, potentially leading to chronic stress, anxiety-related disorders, and a diminished capacity for natural behaviors such as exploration, problem-solving, and social interaction. A horse in this state may lose its natural curiosity and responsiveness, becoming disengaged rather than willing and cooperative. Ethical and science-based training approaches that emphasize positive learning experiences, choice, and clear communication can help prevent learned helplessness, promoting a more trusting and mutually respectful relationship between horse and handler. By recognizing and addressing the signs of learned helplessness in horses, trainers and caregivers can work toward fostering an environment where horses feel safe, empowered, and able to interact with their world in a healthy and adaptive manner.

Ultimately, learned helplessness serves as a stark reminder of the importance of agency, both in humans and animals. Whether in equine training or human psychology, maintaining an internal locus of control is essential for well-being, motivation, and resilience. By creating environments that encourage autonomy and responsiveness rather than suppression and passivity, we can help ensure that both people and horses retain their ability to engage meaningfully with the world around them.

Polyvagal Theory, developed by Dr. Stephen Porges, provides a framework for understanding how the autonomic nervous system (ANS) regulates behavior, emotional states, and social engagement in mammals. This theory is particularly relevant to equine behavior, welfare, and training, as it helps explain how horses perceive and respond to their environment based on autonomic states. At the core of Polyvagal Theory is the idea that the **vagus nerve**, which plays a central role in regulating physiological responses to safety and threat, operates in three distinct branches that correspond to different states of engagement: **the ventral vagal system (social engagement and relaxation), the sympathetic nervous system (mobilization and fight-or-flight), and the dorsal vagal system (immobilization and shutdown).** These states are influenced by **neuroception**, an unconscious process by which the nervous system continuously scans the environment for cues of safety or danger, shaping behavioral responses accordingly.

Horses, as prey animals, rely heavily on neuroception to assess their surroundings and determine whether they should engage socially, flee from a perceived threat, or shut down in response to overwhelming stress. Unlike cognitive perception, which involves conscious awareness, neuroception is an automatic, subcortical process that allows an organism to react before it has time to think. In horses, neuroception is finely tuned to detect minute changes in their environment, including human body language, vocal tones, and the emotional states of those around them. This sensitivity explains why horses often respond to subtle shifts in human intention, posture, or energy before explicit cues are given.

When a horse perceives safety, the **ventral vagal system** is active, allowing for social engagement, curiosity, and learning. This state is characterized by soft eyes, relaxed ears, a rhythmic breath, and an overall willingness to interact. In this mode, the horse can form meaningful connections with humans and other horses, engage in play, and explore new experiences without excessive fear. Training and handling are most effective when the horse is in this autonomic state, as it promotes trust, cognitive flexibility, and a capacity for nuanced learning.

When a horse detects threat, the sympathetic nervous system becomes dominant, activating the fight-or-flight response. This shift is crucial for survival, enabling rapid movement, heightened vigilance, and increased muscle tone to facilitate escape. Signs of sympathetic activation in horses include pricked ears, widened eyes, tension in the jaw and neck, raised head carriage, and rapid breathing. Many traditional training methods rely on triggering this response through pressure, discomfort, or force, assuming that submission follows from exerting dominance. However, if the horse remains in this heightened state for too long without an opportunity to return to safety, the nervous system can become dysregulated, leading to chronic stress, anxiety-related behaviors, and difficulty learning.

If a horse perceives that escape or resistance is impossible, the **dorsal vagal system**, associated with **immobilization and shutdown**, becomes dominant. This state is the physiological foundation of **learned helplessness**, where the horse ceases to respond to stimuli because previous attempts to act or escape have been futile. Horses in this state often display signs of **dissociation**, such as a dull or vacant stare, a lowered head, decreased responsiveness, and a lack of engagement with their surroundings. To an untrained observer, these horses may appear calm or obedient, but they are in a state of **biological conservation**, suppressing movement and emotion as a last-resort survival mechanism. The dorsal vagal response is an adaptive function when escape is not possible, but when repeatedly activated through aversive training methods, confinement, or neglect, it can lead to long-term physiological and psychological distress.

Understanding **neuroception** and **Polyvagal Theory** provides invaluable insights into how we can create environments and training approaches that support a horse's nervous system in maintaining **ventral vagal engagement** rather than chronic sympathetic arousal or dorsal vagal shutdown. Training approaches that promote **co-regulation**, the ability of the nervous system to attune to another being's state, are particularly beneficial. Because horses are deeply sensitive to human nervous system states, a dysregulated or tense handler can inadvertently trigger sympathetic activation in the horse. Conversely, a human who embodies calmness, presence, and rhythmic breathing can help the horse shift toward a state of social engagement and relaxation.

Practical applications of Polyvagal Theory in horse training emphasize trust-based methods, choice, and autonomy over dominance-based approaches. Using gradual progression, clear communication, and non-threatening body language fosters an environment where the horse's neuroception continually receives signals of safety. Practices such as slow, deliberate movement, rhythmic breathing, and mutual awareness can encourage **ventral vagal engagement**, facilitating learning and deepening the horse-human bond. Conversely, abrupt movements, harsh tones, or unpredictable pressure can activate **sympathetic or**

dorsal vagal responses, making learning more difficult and increasing stress-related behaviors such as bolting, head-tossing, or freezing.

By integrating Polyvagal Theory into equine care, we can move beyond outdated paradigms of force and compliance, recognizing that a horse's behavioral responses are deeply rooted in autonomic function rather than willful disobedience. This perspective allows for a more compassionate, neuroscience-based approach to horse training and management, prioritizing emotional well-being alongside physical health. A horse that feels safe—one whose neuroception consistently registers its environment as non-threatening, will not only be easier to train but will also experience greater well-being, forming relationships based on mutual trust rather than conditioned submission. While widely influential in therapeutic and trauma-informed care, some critics argue that the Polyvagal Theory lacks direct empirical support in some areas and that its integration into broader neuroscientific frameworks is still evolving. Nonetheless, its conceptual contributions have transformed approaches to understanding the autonomic nervous system in relational and clinical contexts.

Trigger stacking is a phenomenon in which multiple stressors accumulate over a short period, amplifying a horse's stress response and potentially leading to an exaggerated reaction that seems disproportionate to any single trigger. Borrowed from the field of dog training, this concept highlights how stressors, when stacked without adequate recovery time, can overwhelm an animal's nervous system, making it difficult for them to regulate their arousal and return to a baseline state of calm. In horses, which are highly attuned to their environment and rely on rapid assessments of safety or danger, trigger stacking can significantly impact behavior, learning, and overall welfare.

Horses, as prey animals, have evolved to respond quickly to perceived threats, often defaulting to flight, fight, or freeze behaviors when faced with stressors. However, when stress accumulates too quickly without an opportunity for recovery, the nervous system can become dysregulated, leading to heightened reactivity or, conversely, a shutdown response. For example, a horse that encounters an unfamiliar environment, a loud noise, and abrupt handling in quick succession may react explosively, whereas any one of these stressors in isolation may not have caused a significant response. This is because each stressor incrementally raises the horse's sympathetic arousal level, reducing its ability to regulate and making it more prone to a fight-or-flight reaction.

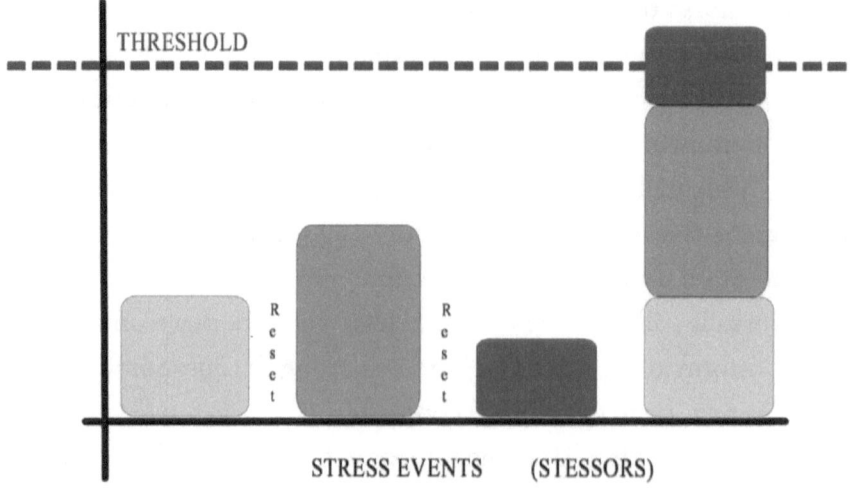

At the neurophysiological level, trigger stacking is deeply connected to the functioning of the autonomic nervous system (ANS). The **sympathetic nervous system**, responsible for mobilization in response to threats, triggers the release of stress hormones such as cortisol and norepinephrine. If the horse does not have time to recover and engage the **parasympathetic nervous system**, which restores calm and homeostasis, stress continues to build, making the animal increasingly reactive. This process is exacerbated by the way neuroreceptors regulate stress responses. The **upregulation and downregulation of neuroreceptors** influence how cells respond to neurochemical signals, affecting a horse's sensitivity to stress over time. Cellular upregulation and downregulation are fundamental biological processes that allow cells to adjust their responsiveness to external stimuli, maintaining balance and adaptability in various physiological systems. **Upregulation** occurs when a cell increases the number or sensitivity of its receptors, proteins, or enzymes in response to reduced stimulation. This allows the cell to become more sensitive to a signal that has been diminished or absent. For example, when neurotransmitter levels drop in the brain, neurons may upregulate receptor expression to enhance their ability to detect the remaining signal. This mechanism plays a crucial role in neuroplasticity, learning, and adaptation. Similarly, muscle cells upregulate glucose transporters (GLUT4) in response to exercise, improving glucose uptake and energy efficiency.

Conversely, **downregulation** occurs when cells reduce the number or sensitivity of receptors to prevent overstimulation. This is often seen in cases of prolonged exposure to high hormone or neurotransmitter levels, such as chronic stress leading to the downregulation of glucocorticoid receptors, reducing the body's ability to regulate stress over time. A well-known example of downregulation occurs in drug tolerance, where repeated use of opioids or other addictive substances leads to a decrease in receptor availability, requiring higher doses to achieve the same effect. Similarly, in insulin resistance, prolonged high insulin levels lead to downregulation of insulin receptors, making cells less responsive to insulin and contributing to insulin resistance in horses.

These regulatory mechanisms are crucial for homeostasis, protecting the body from excessive stimulation while ensuring cells remain responsive when needed. In Neuroendocrinology, they influence hormone sensitivity, affecting everything from metabolism to reproductive health. In neuroscience, they shape learning, memory, and addiction by modulating synaptic strength. Overall, these cellular processes exemplify the body's ability to dynamically adjust to its environment, ensuring optimal function and survival.

The amygdala, central to processing emotions and fear responses, becomes hyperactive during repeated stress exposure. When trigger stacking occurs, the amygdala's activation increases, making the horse more likely to react defensively. In contrast, cortical areas and their connections such as the frontal lobe, cingulate cortex, and premotor regions play a role in regulating responses and enabling adaptive behavior. If the horse is given sufficient recovery time between stressors, these regulatory areas can engage effectively, allowing the animal to assess situations more rationally rather than reacting impulsively.

The effects of trigger stacking vary between individuals; some horses have a lower threshold for accumulated stress and may become overwhelmed more easily than others. Recognizing the signs of trigger stacking, such as increased tension, escalating flight responses, difficulty focusing, or sudden outbursts, is crucial for handlers and trainers. A key strategy for preventing stress escalation is allowing the horse's nervous system to **pendulate**, or oscillate between heightened arousal and relaxation, ensuring that recovery occurs before another stressor is introduced. This natural rhythm of arousal and regulation fosters emotional resilience and helps horses develop more adaptive responses to stress.

From a practical standpoint, preventing trigger stacking in training and handling requires an approach that prioritizes predictability, choice, and controlled exposure to stimuli. For instance, gradually desensitizing a horse to a new environment while allowing frequent breaks to process and regulate will be far more effective than overwhelming the animal with multiple stressors in a short period.

The cardiac nervous system operates in close communication with **baroreceptors** and **chemoreceptors**, which continuously monitor the horse's internal physiological state. **Baroreceptors**, located in the walls of blood vessels, detect changes in blood pressure and trigger compensatory adjustments in heart rate and vascular resistance. **Chemoreceptors**, on the other hand, assess oxygen and carbon dioxide levels in the bloodstream, ensuring that the heart's output is dynamically adjusted to meet the body's metabolic demands. These sensory feedback mechanisms allow horses to sustain high-intensity exertion while maintaining cardiovascular efficiency, a trait that makes them exceptional endurance and performance athletes.

However, stress plays a significant role in modulating the cardiac nervous system, affecting the balance between sympathetic and parasympathetic activity. **Acute stress**, such as a sudden environmental change or a perceived threat, results in an immediate SNS response, rapid heart rate elevation and increased cardiac output to prepare the horse for action. While this is a normal and adaptive function, chronic stress or poor welfare conditions can dysregulate this balance, leading to prolonged SNS activation without sufficient PNS recovery. Over time, **autonomic imbalance** can contribute to **arrhythmias, reduced cardiac efficiency, immune suppression**, and heightened susceptibility to disease. This highlights the importance of maintaining a low-stress environment and ensuring horses experience adequate periods of relaxation and recovery to support cardiac health.

The equine heart is uniquely adapted for athletic performance, capable of rapidly increasing its output through sympathetic stimulation. This ability enables horses to sustain powerful bursts of speed, making them one of the most physiologically remarkable land mammals in terms of cardiovascular efficiency. Just as important, however, is the parasympathetic system's ability to facilitate rapid recovery after exertion, efficiently restoring heart rate, regulating metabolic processes, and preventing exercise-induced cardiac strain. The interplay between these two autonomic branches determines not only a horse's performance capacity but also its resilience to stress and its long-term cardiovascular well-being.

Understanding the cardiac nervous system has far-reaching implications for equine training, veterinary medicine, and welfare. By monitoring **HRV**, trainers can assess a horse's ability to cope with training stress, refine conditioning programs, and detect early signs of overtraining or autonomic dysfunction. Advances in equine cardiology continue to improve our ability to diagnose and manage heart conditions, optimize performance, and develop science-based **best practices** for handling, training, and overall horse care.

The Window of Tolerance, a concept introduced by Daniel Siegel, provides a valuable framework for understanding how horses process emotions, integrate sensory information, and develop resilience in managing stress. This window represents the optimal range within which a horse can experience arousal or stress without becoming overwhelmed, allowing for learning, neuroplasticity, and behavioral adaptability. When a horse operates within this range, it can engage in training, problem-solving, and social interactions while maintaining emotional balance. However, when pushed beyond the limits of its window of tolerance, a horse may experience dysregulation, leading to either hyperarousal, manifesting as heightened vigilance, flight, or defensive aggression or hypoarousal, where the horse shuts down, disengages, or "freezes."

Horses, as prey animals, have highly sensitive nervous systems finely tuned for survival. Some horses, particularly those with a history of trauma or heightened sensitivity, may have a narrower window of tolerance, making them more prone to stress-induced reactions. When exposed to overwhelming stimuli, such as unpredictable handling, excessive pressure, or environmental stressors, they can be pushed into sympathetic over-arousal. In this state, the autonomic nervous system triggers a fight-or-flight response, inhibiting cognitive engagement and making learning nearly impossible. Alternatively, if stress is prolonged or inescapable, a horse may enter a dorsal vagal shutdown, a protective state characterized by passivity, learned helplessness, or a lack of responsiveness.

Effective training involves skillfully guiding a horse to the very edges of its window of tolerance without exceeding them. By introducing manageable levels of challenge and allowing the horse to process mild stress while maintaining a sense of safety, we encourage the development of new neural connections, promote focus, and reinforce positive coping mechanisms. This approach, known as **pendulation**, involves intentional cycles of stress exposure followed by recovery, allowing the nervous system to oscillate between states of arousal and relaxation. Such rhythmic fluctuations help to reduce **allostatic load** (the accumulated physiological burden of stress) and gradually expand the horse's capacity for emotional and physiological regulation. Unlike desensitization techniques that may flood the nervous system with excessive stimuli, controlled stress exposure followed by relief strengthens resilience, enhances problem-solving abilities, and fosters a sense of agency in the horse.

It is important to recognize that staying too comfortably within the window of tolerance without challenge can lead to stagnation, shrinking the horse's capacity to cope with new experiences. Conversely, overexposure to stress, particularly without adequate recovery, can result in trauma and maladaptive behaviors. The key to expanding the window lies in carefully pacing experiences, offering predictability and safety, and ensuring that moments of discomfort are paired with successful resolution. Handlers who can read subtle shifts in equine body language, such as changes in breath rate, muscle tension, ear positioning, and eye expression, can effectively gauge when a horse is nearing the edges of its tolerance and adjust accordingly.

Expanding a horse's window of tolerance is not only beneficial for performance but also for overall welfare. A horse that learns to experience stress without immediate reactivity gains confidence, emotional stability, and a greater ability to regulate itself in novel situations. By fostering neuroplasticity (the brain's ability to reorganize and form new neural pathways) this approach supports cognitive flexibility and adaptive behavior, ensuring the horse can navigate challenges with curiosity rather than fear. The end goal is not just compliance but true emotional regulation, where the horse remains present and aware of its options even in moments of stress.

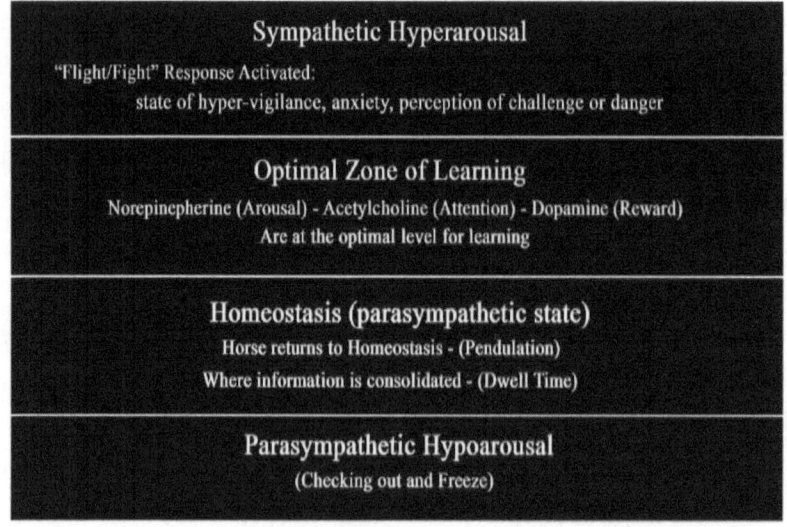

In summary, a thoughtful understanding of the window of tolerance enables equine professionals to train with empathy, structure experiences that promote resilience, and create horses that are both mentally and emotionally sound. By working within and gradually expanding this window, we help horses cultivate adaptability, reduce anxiety-driven behaviors, and develop a robust nervous system capable of handling life's challenges.

The Yerkes-Dodson Law describes the relationship between arousal levels and performance, emphasizing that optimal learning and performance occur at moderate levels of arousal. If arousal is too low, engagement and responsiveness diminish; if it is too high, cognitive function and the ability to process information become impaired. This principle is particularly relevant when considering horse behavior and training. For a horse to learn effectively, it must be in an optimal state of alertness, attentive but not anxious, engaged but not overwhelmed. A horse that is too relaxed may appear disinterested or unresponsive to training cues, while one that is overstimulated may struggle to process new information and react with fear or avoidance.

From a neurobiological perspective, this balance is governed by the release of key neurotransmitters such as dopamine, norepinephrine, and acetylcholine, which play essential roles in attention, learning, and memory consolidation. When a horse is in an optimal arousal state, these neurotransmitters support focus and retention of new information. However, excessive stress activates the amygdala (the brain's center for processing fear) and triggers the release of high levels of cortisol, the stress hormone. This not only impairs cognitive function but also increases the likelihood of fear-based reactions, which can be counterproductive to training and may lead to undesirable behaviors such as flight responses, freezing, or defensive aggression.

Applying the **Yerkes-Dodson Law** in horse training requires careful management of arousal levels through thoughtful, structured exposure to challenges. Trainers and handlers can achieve this by using gradual desensitization, clear communication, and well-timed and consistent reinforcement. Introducing new stimuli in a controlled manner allows the horse to build confidence without triggering an excessive stress response. Likewise, maintaining consistency in training methods and ensuring that expectations remain clear can help prevent frustration and anxiety. By keeping a horse within its **optimal learning zone**, trainers can enhance their ability to retain information, build trust, and develop resilience to new or potentially stressful situations.

The **Orienting Response (OR)** in horses is a fundamental psychophysiological mechanism that allows horses to detect and respond to changes in their environment. This response is essential for survival, enabling the horse to assess potential threats and make rapid decisions about whether to react or remain at ease. When a stimulus, such as a sudden noise or an unexpected movement carries high significance, the OR is pronounced, directing the horse's attention toward the source of the disturbance. However, when the stimulus is perceived as insignificant or non-threatening, the OR gradually diminishes, allowing the horse to conserve energy and maintain a state of calm.

At the core of this response is the **Reticular Activating System (RAS)**, which plays a pivotal role in detecting imbalances in homeostasis. Sensory receptors throughout the horse's body relay information to the RAS, which then communicates with the **thalamus** to process and filter the stimulus. Once evaluated, the information is sent to the motor system, triggering an appropriate action, whether it be an alert stance, investigative behavior, or swift movement away from potential danger. This intricate system ensures that horses can respond effectively to changes in their surroundings, restoring equilibrium with minimal disruption. Importantly, when given the freedom to process stimuli without interference, horses are remarkably adept at returning to a balanced state on their own.

Additionally, predictability and expectancy play crucial roles in the horse's cognitive framework. A stable and predictable environment fosters a sense of security, reducing unnecessary OR activation and preventing heightened vigilance. When horses can anticipate their surroundings, they are less prone to stress and reactivity, allowing for more efficient energy management and overall well-being.

Trauma and Fear Conditioning

Horses, like humans, can carry the imprint of trauma long after the original event has passed. Even years after experiencing a frightening or painful event, horses may continue to display defensive behaviors rooted in their past experiences. These conditioned responses can become automatic, even in safe environments, if the surroundings or specific stimuli resemble the context of the original trauma. This occurs because trauma fundamentally alters the nervous system, often leading to a persistent state of hyperarousal in which the horse perceives the world through a heightened lens of risk and a diminished sense of safety. Societal normalization of certain training practices or forms of neglect can obscure the recognition of these trauma-induced behaviors, making it difficult to identify and address the underlying issues effectively.

When a horse experiences a traumatic event, its brain encodes a complex array of sensory and physiological signals through the reticular activating system (RAS). These signals include changes in heart rate, breathing, sympathetic nervous system activation, and gastrointestinal function. The brain integrates these sensations with the context of the event, forming strong associative memories that link specific environmental cues to the experience. In future encounters with similar stimuli, the brain rapidly runs a predictive simulation, triggering the same physiological and emotional responses as if the original trauma were happening again. Over time, these repeated associations shape the horse's internal model of the world, significantly influencing its behavioral responses to perceived threats and safety cues.

Dissociation is another significant neurobiological response to trauma, often manifesting as a shutdown or tonic immobility in horses. This occurs when a horse is overwhelmed by a threat that it cannot escape or fight. While the exact mechanisms of dissociation are still being explored, neuroimaging studies suggest that it involves a functional disconnection within the cortical-limbic system, particularly affecting the amygdala and anterior cingulate cortex. This disruption dampens emotional and interoceptive awareness, effectively reducing the horse's ability to process sensory and emotional inputs. While dissociation serves as an adaptive survival mechanism, allowing the horse to endure extreme stress, it can lead to long-term behavioral consequences, such as learned helplessness, where the horse appears emotionally shut down and unresponsive to its surroundings.

Fear conditioning plays a critical role in how horses respond to perceived threats. The amygdala is central to this process, activating various brain regions responsible for coordinating the fear response.

When a horse encounters a fear-inducing stimulus, the central nucleus of the amygdala signals the periaqueductal gray in the midbrain, producing the classic freezing response, a common reaction in prey animals assessing potential danger. While activation of the lateral hypothalamus triggers the sympathetic nervous system, increasing heart rate and arousal in preparation for fight or flight. Additionally, the amygdala's interaction with the locus coeruleus, a region responsible for norepinephrine production, heightens vigilance, making the horse acutely aware of its environment. These neural circuits ensure that horses respond swiftly to threats, but they also explain why fear memories are so persistent once a fear response is conditioned, it can be difficult to extinguish.

A single traumatic event can trigger long-term potentiation (LTP) in a horse's brain, creating a lasting memory of fear or aversion. When a horse experiences a sudden, intense stressor such as a painful mishap, a frightening encounter, or an overwhelming sensory overload, the amygdala and hippocampus rapidly encode the event. The amygdala, responsible for processing fear, signals the release of stress hormones like cortisol and adrenaline, heightening the horse's state of alertness. Simultaneously, glutamate release in the hippocampus strengthens synaptic connections through NMDA receptor activation, facilitating LTP. This synaptic reinforcement means that even a single exposure to the trauma can result in a long-lasting, hypersensitive response to similar stimuli in the future. The next time the horse encounters a related situation whether it be a certain location, object, or sensory cue, the potentiated neural circuits react with heightened reactivity, often leading to flight, freeze, or defensive behavior. Unlike humans, who can rationalize fears, horses rely on associative learning, meaning that one powerful experience can establish a deeply ingrained response pattern that is difficult to extinguish without deliberate, careful desensitization and counterconditioning.

Understanding Self-Preservation in the Horse: The Neuroscience of Fear and Motivation

Horses, as prey animals, are neurologically hardwired to evaluate their surroundings with exceptional speed and precision, continually scanning for potential threats. This capacity for rapid threat assessment, shaped by millions of years of evolution, remains deeply embedded in their nervous system. While humans often view horses as companions, athletes, or working partners, the horse's brain is still shaped by its evolutionary past, instinctively categorizing other beings—including humans—as either safe or threatening. This survival-driven lens profoundly influences their behavioral responses and learning processes.

Selective breeding over centuries has refined traits such as size, conformation, temperament, and even intelligence, but the fundamental instinct for self-preservation remains unchanged. This primal drive is a key factor in both the horse's trainability and its occasional resistance to human cues. Even though humans are not predators in the conventional sense, behaviors such as abrupt movements, loud vocalizations, or sustained direct eye contact can activate a horse's survival circuits, triggering autonomic arousal and defensive reactions.

From a neuroendocrinological standpoint, a horse's perception of threat initiates a cascade through the hypothalamic-pituitary-adrenal (HPA) axis, resulting in cortisol release and a surge of physiological adjustments designed to enhance survival—elevated heart rate, increased muscle tone, and sharpened sensory awareness. This system, mediated by neurotransmitters such as norepinephrine and dopamine, also guides the horse's natural drive to seek relief and safety. Training techniques like pressure and release are effective because they leverage this neurobiology: the removal of pressure activates dopamine pathways associated with reward and reinforces the behavior that led to relief, making learning clear and efficient.

However, a common error in horsemanship is to treat horses as though they are mechanical entities expected to respond with uniform precision to equipment or cues. Horses are sentient, emotionally complex animals whose responses are shaped by prior experiences, current sensory input, and emotional states governed largely by the limbic system—particularly the amygdala, which processes fear and threat detection. In training, horses often move fluidly between states of suspicion and curiosity, reflecting the interplay between norepinephrine-driven arousal (heightened alertness) and dopamine-driven motivation (approach and reward).

While tools and cues can reliably shape behavior, they do not override a horse's core survival instincts. A horse may tolerate discomfort out of necessity, but it will resist or attempt to escape overwhelming fear. Mild anxiety can be an effective motivator, helping the horse focus on problem-solving and learning. Yet, when fear escalates to panic, the horse's cognitive processing degrades. Higher-order structures such as the cingulate cortex—responsible for emotional regulation and nuanced decision-making—become less active, and the horse defaults to reflexive, instinctual reactions. Unfortunately, these behaviors are often misinterpreted by humans as stubbornness or irrationality, when they are in fact manifestations of deeply rooted neurobiological processes.

Respecting and managing a horse's fear threshold is therefore critical. Clarity, consistency, and the provision of sufficient time to process new stimuli can make the difference between a positive learning experience and a traumatic one. Just as humans struggle to make rational choices under extreme threat, horses overwhelmed by fear are neurologically incapable of learning or cooperating effectively. When given adequate space, time, and a sense of security, their nervous system can downregulate, shifting from norepinephrine-driven hyperarousal to an oxytocin-supported state of calm, connection, and trust.

Ultimately, effective horsemanship depends on understanding and working within the horse's natural neurobiology. Building trust-based partnerships, rather than relying on fear-driven compliance, aligns with how the equine brain processes information, stress, and safety. When confronted with a frightened horse, the most effective approach is often to provide the same reassurance and patience we would extend to a frightened human—creating an environment where the nervous system can settle, and true learning can occur.

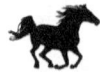

Autonomy and Self Reliance

"The more we learn about the horse's brain, the more we realize that the best training is not about control—it's about conversation."

—Dr. Stephen Peters

Horses, like other cognitively complex animals, thrive when given the opportunity to make choices and influence their own environment within safe and well-structured boundaries. Autonomy does not mean permissiveness—it means recognizing that the horse's nervous system is built to assess, adapt, and learn through experience. When horses are allowed to participate in decision-making, even in small ways, it activates key neural systems involved in cognition and emotional regulation. Though the equine frontal cortex is less elaborated than that of a human, it still plays a central role in processing novelty, inhibiting impulsive responses, and integrating sensory information. The cingulate cortex supports behavioral flexibility and error correction, while the basal ganglia contribute to habit formation and motor sequencing. When we engage these systems through training that supports autonomy, we promote neuroplastic changes that build confidence, cognitive resilience, and emotional stability.

This approach aligns with the Five Domains model of equine welfare, particularly the domain of mental state. Horses that have opportunities for choice and control experience more positive affective states, greater engagement with their environment, and a reduced likelihood of developing stress-induced behavioral problems. On the other hand, when horses are micromanaged—overdirected, overcorrected, or deprived of agency—their behavioral repertoire narrows. They may become anxious, withdrawn, or reactive. Neuroscientifically, this pattern reflects chronic activation of the amygdala, prolonged engagement of the hypothalamic-pituitary-adrenal (HPA) axis, and a dominance of sympathetic arousal over parasympathetic regulation. Over time, this compromises not only behavior but also immune function, digestive health, and learning capacity.

Emotional regulation—the ability to tolerate, recover from, and adapt to stress—develops through experience. Horses that are gradually exposed to manageable stressors, followed by restoration of safety and calm, build robust connections between the frontal cortex, limbic regions, and autonomic control centers. These connections underlie self-regulatory behavior. Rather than reacting reflexively to every novel stimulus, the horse learns to pause, assess, and respond. This mirrors the concept of stress inoculation found in human psychology: resilience is not built by avoiding stress but by learning how to navigate it effectively. When a horse hesitates in front of an unfamiliar object, it is not disobeying—it is engaging its internal regulatory mechanisms. Allowing space for this process reinforces cognitive, rather than reactive, circuits.

The autonomic nervous system plays a critical role in this regulation. During moments of challenge or alertness, sympathetic arousal drives energy mobilization and heightened vigilance. This is adaptive—but only if followed by a return to parasympathetic balance.

The parasympathetic branch facilitates rest, digestion, and social engagement. Horses trained to self-regulate are more adept at moving fluidly between these states. Behavioral indicators of this shift include licking, chewing, blinking, head-lowering, and yawning. These signals are not trivial—they reflect meaningful physiological transitions. Yawning, for example, is linked to shifts in autonomic tone, possibly involving hypothalamic and brainstem regulation of arousal, thermoregulation, and social bonding. It may be influenced by neuroendocrine changes such as decreases in cortisol or increases in oxytocin and serotonin. Still, context matters: repetitive yawning may also signal discomfort, gastrointestinal tension, or frustration, requiring careful interpretation.

Allowing horses opportunities for decision-making—such as choosing a route on a ride or approaching a novel object at their own pace—stimulates dopaminergic circuits involved in reward, motivation, and curiosity. These include pathways connecting the ventral tegmental area to the nucleus accumbens, systems that support approach behavior and promote cognitive engagement. Structured choices, introduced in controlled settings, help horses learn that they can influence their environment, building behavioral flexibility and trust. These moments of agency are not just training tools; they are exercises in shaping the brain. They reinforce circuits that allow horses to remain curious under pressure, rather than shutting down or reacting defensively.

Some handlers equate obedience with reliability and dependence with safety, but over-reliance on constant direction may undermine a horse's ability to problem-solve or recover emotionally in dynamic environments. Just as human children mature through carefully scaffolded independence, horses develop their cognitive and emotional capacities when given the right amount of freedom, paired with consistency and clarity. Gradual exposure to novelty, combined with positive reinforcement and calm leadership, supports the development of acetylcholine-mediated attention networks, enabling horses to focus, process, and recover more efficiently. Linking specific cues—such as a verbal signal or a rider's exhale—with states of calm further reinforces associative learning and builds anchors for emotional recovery in future stressful situations.

Horses that have been given the opportunity to think, assess, and choose tend to respond with greater clarity and control under pressure. Rather than relying exclusively on external direction, they access internally built systems of regulation supported by functional connections between the limbic system and the prefrontal cortex. In moments of challenge, they don't freeze or flee automatically; they process. This neurobiological confidence is visible in their behavior—calm eyes, measured movement, and an ability to engage with the environment even when aroused.

Ultimately, fostering autonomy in horses is not about relinquishing leadership; it's about refining it. A horse that feels safe enough to think, confident enough to explore, and supported enough to regulate its own internal state is not just compliant—it is engaged. These horses are more reliable, more adaptable, and more expressive. The result is a deeper, more responsive partnership built not on dominance but on shared experience, co-regulation, and mutual trust.

Legendary horseman Tom Dorrance encapsulated the essence of cultivating internal agency in horses, emphasizing: *"The thing you are trying to help the horse do is to use his own mind. You are trying to present something and then let him figure out how to get there."* This philosophy aligns closely with promoting an internal locus of control, empowering the horse neurologically, cognitively, and emotionally to engage meaningfully with its environment.

SECTION III

Learning, Training, and Welfare

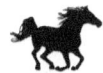

Learning, Memory, and Training

"Real teaching and real learning happen when you're listening closely enough to answer the horse's questions."
—Dr. Stephen Peters

Learning and memory in horses are governed by sophisticated neurobiological processes, deeply influenced by neuroplasticity—the brain's remarkable ability to reorganize and strengthen neural connections in response to experience. Optimal learning occurs under conditions of moderate arousal, characterized by the balanced release of dopamine, norepinephrine, and acetylcholine, neurotransmitters essential for attention, memory formation, and behavioral flexibility. However, excessive arousal—often triggered by fear or stress—activates the amygdala and triggers defensive reactions (fight, flight, or freeze), severely compromising the horse's capacity to learn. Thus, a state of "relaxed alertness," in which a horse is engaged yet calm and secure, is crucial for optimal cognitive functioning and effective memory consolidation.

Sympathetic arousal plays a pivotal role in learning by enhancing attention and facilitating neuroplasticity through controlled releases of norepinephrine and acetylcholine. Dopamine, peaking at optimal arousal, reinforces successful behaviors and motivates continued engagement. Conversely, keeping horses overly comfortable and unchallenged limits engagement and shrinks their comfort zone, making them increasingly reactive and anxious when exposed to novel stimuli. Expanding a horse's comfort zone through gradual exposure to new stimuli—termed pendulation—alternates between manageable sympathetic arousal and parasympathetic recovery, building resilience and confidence. Training strategies that completely avoid stress may create short-term comfort but fail to develop the neural pathways necessary for managing future stress, ultimately impairing a horse's adaptability and cognitive growth.

Working memory serves as the entry point for new information, but its capacity is limited and easily overwhelmed by distractions. Horses, evolved as prey animals, possess heightened vigilance; sudden sensory stimuli rapidly capture attention, activating the amygdala and releasing stress hormones like norepinephrine and cortisol, disrupting hippocampal functions and impairing memory formation. Trainers can enhance learning by managing sensory input, improving the signal-to-noise ratio through clear, precise, and consistent cues. Associative learning, facilitated by glutamate-mediated synaptic plasticity (especially long-term potentiation), integrates new experiences into long-term memory, while dopamine signals reinforce behaviors that yield rewards, leading to increased cognitive flexibility and efficient learning through incremental shaping and targeted reinforcement.

The basal ganglia, particularly the striatum, play a central role in habit formation and skill automation. Initially, new behaviors require active cognitive engagement from the frontal cortex, but through repetition, control shifts to the basal ganglia, optimizing behavior execution with minimal conscious effort—a state known as hypofrontality. Dopamine release from the substantia nigra reinforces successful actions, strengthening neural pathways. Clear and consistent training allows the basal ganglia to form reliable neural patterns, facilitating rapid skill acquisition and fluid behavior. Conversely, inconsistent training weakens neural associations, leading to confusion and slower learning.

Reward prediction error (RPE) significantly influences equine learning. Unexpected rewards cause dopamine surges (positive RPE), reinforcing behavior, whereas predictable rewards result in diminished dopamine response (zero RPE), leading to disengagement during repetitive tasks. Negative RPE, when anticipated rewards fail to appear, weakens learned associations. Thus, variable reinforcement, incorporating elements of surprise and challenge, maintains dopamine engagement and enhances motivation and adaptive problem-solving abilities, compared to monotonous repetition.

Curiosity and exploration stimulate hippocampal neuroplasticity through dopamine release, enhancing memory formation and engagement. However, memory consolidation, the stabilization of short-term into long-term memories, primarily occurs during sleep, facilitated by acetylcholine. Allowing periods of rest following training optimizes memory retention and ensures stable learning.

Timing, rhythm, and synchrony significantly influence communication and learning between horse and rider. Horses naturally respond to rhythmic stimuli, deeply embedded through evolutionary neuroethology. Achieving synchrony requires patience, observation, and precise timing, enhancing clear neural pathways and motor neuron myelination. Tension disrupts synchronization, emphasizing the importance of relaxed, rhythmic interactions. Riders should practice aligning their movements and breathing patterns with their horses, leveraging natural herd instincts and the basal ganglia's capacity for automating synchronized movements.

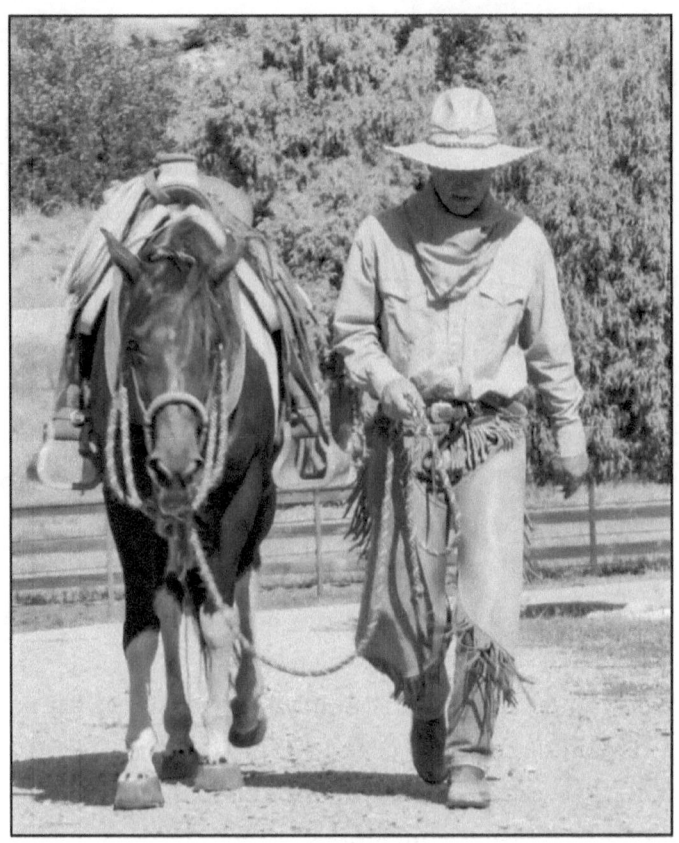

Behaviorism, originally focusing solely on observable behavior and external reinforcement, has evolved to incorporate cognitive, emotional, and neurobiological insights. Understanding horses' cognitive processes, emotional states, and sensory perceptions enriches traditional conditioning methods, fostering deeper connections and more humane training practices. Classical and operant conditioning remain foundational, but modern training recognizes the significance of cognitive engagement, intrinsic motivation, and emotional balance. Ethical horse training integrates these perspectives, prioritizing welfare and cognitive enrichment alongside behavioral compliance.

Operant conditioning, involving reinforcement and punishment, has historically dominated training methodologies. However, effective equine learning involves both operant conditioning and cognitive exploration—activities driven by curiosity and intrinsic motivation. Encouraging horses to actively engage and problem-solve fosters deeper, more meaningful learning experiences than mere compliance to external stimuli.

The International Society for Equitation Science (ISES) outlines ten scientifically grounded training principles emphasizing safety, welfare, clarity, and respect for equine mental and emotional states. These principles advocate systematic desensitization, ethical use of reinforcement, and structured training steps. Aligning training practices with ISES principles ensures clear communication, reduces stress, enhances learning efficiency, and promotes overall equine welfare.

Neuroscientifically, understanding pressure and relief is essential for effective training. Relief is more than stopping pressure; it involves transitioning from sympathetic arousal to parasympathetic calm, mediated by neurotransmitters like oxytocin and serotonin. Effective training consistently facilitates this physiological shift, ensuring that learning occurs without residual stress or anxiety.

Habituation and desensitization (gradual neural adaptation) reduce excessive responses through controlled, repetitive, low-stress exposure. Unlike flooding, which can cause panic and psychological trauma, gradual adaptation preserves horses' natural sensitivity, building confidence and resilience without dulling their responsiveness.

Ultimately, a holistic, multidisciplinary approach—integrating behavioral science, cognitive neuroscience, ethology, and welfare principles—provides the most comprehensive and humane training model. This approach prioritizes understanding of the horse's nervous system, cognitive engagement, emotional resilience, intrinsic motivation, and effective, ethically driven behavior modification, ensuring not only performance excellence but enhanced welfare and psychological well-being in horses.

"In Step"
by Dr. Stephen Peters

There is a rhythm in the horse
that isn't taught,
only felt—
in the sway of a walk,
the lift of a trot,
the quiet of a shared breath.

The horse does not seek to lead or follow—
only to *be* in time,
to move with what is true
and feel the weight of presence balanced,
light as a whisper on the back.

When we carry ourselves with balance,
they adjust their own.
When our signals are quiet and consistent,
they soften and listen.
Their bodies respond in moments—
to breath, to posture,
to the space we give or take.

They're always seeking rhythm,
even when we disrupt it.
Always willing
to return to center
if we'll meet them there.

But when we rush, or freeze, or grasp too tight—
when our minds wander or our hands demand—
the rhythm falters.
The dance is lost.

Yet still,
the horse waits.
Soft-eyed, listening,
ready to begin again.
Willing to meet us
where movement becomes music,
and silence,
a shared note of understanding.

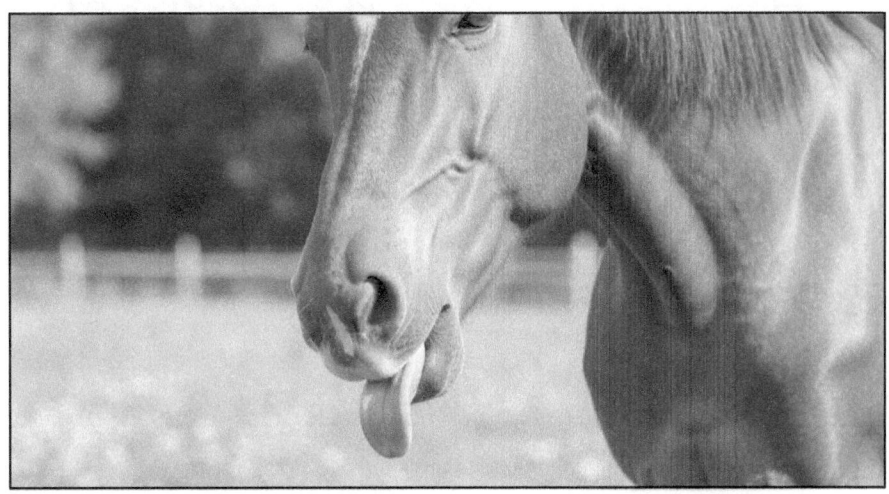

"Turn them out when they're going good and they come back better."

—Tom Dorrance

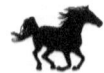

Environment, Welfare, and the Five Domains Model

"Welfare isn't just physical comfort—it's room for curiosity, connection, expression, and a nervous system at ease."

—Dr. Stephen Peters

The Five Domains of Equine Welfare: A Contemporary Approach to Improving Horse Well-being

Promoting equine welfare involves much more than simply preventing pain or discomfort; it demands a proactive commitment to enhancing the overall quality of life for horses. The Five Domains Model, introduced by Professor David Mellor and his colleagues, offers a comprehensive approach that incorporates both the physical and mental dimensions of welfare. Unlike previous frameworks such as the Five Freedoms—which mainly aimed at avoiding negative experiences—

the Five Domains Model emphasizes the importance of encouraging positive states and experiences.

Central to this model is the recognition that a horse's emotional and psychological well-being is equally as critical as its physical health. It assesses welfare across five core domains: Nutrition, Physical Environment, Health, Behavioral Interactions, and Mental State. By using these principles, veterinarians, trainers, and horse caretakers can design management practices tailored to meet both the physiological and emotional/psychological needs of horses. This proactive approach strives to create environments where horses can thrive.

Nutrition: More Than Just Feeding

Under the first domain, Nutrition, the focus extends beyond merely providing adequate food; it emphasizes delivering species-appropriate nutrition that fully addresses horses' physiological and metabolic requirements. Horses have evolved for continuous forage intake, thriving on fiber-rich diets primarily composed of hay and pasture. Such diets are crucial for maintaining optimal gut health and mitigating the risk of metabolic disorders. Feeding practices must mirror their natural grazing behaviors to reduce stress, prevent digestive disturbances, and minimize conditions like gastric ulcers. Additionally, uninterrupted access to fresh, clean water is essential, as dehydration poses serious health risks. When horses are fed in group environments, careful oversight is necessary to manage social dynamics and prevent resource guarding behaviors, stress, or nutritional imbalances resulting from dominant herd members limiting food access.

Physical Environment: Creating Safe and Natural Spaces

The second domain of equine welfare, Physical Environment, is vital for ensuring both the comfort and psychological health of horses. An optimal living space must offer protection from extreme weather conditions, including adequate shelter from harsh sun, wind, rain, and cold. At the same time, the design of housing areas should facilitate natural equine behaviors such as lying down, rolling, grazing, and socializing, promoting both physical health and mental stimulation. Horses require ample space that enables unrestricted movement and exploration of their environment, essential for maintaining muscular, skeletal, and joint health. Clean, secure footing is crucial to minimize the risk of slips, falls, or other injuries, while comfortable bedding aids in joint support and provides conditions favorable for rest and recovery. Social interaction is particularly significant, as horses are inherently herd animals that rely on group dynamics for emotional security and stress reduction. Social housing arrangements, therefore, are preferable to solitary confinement, which can lead to loneliness, anxiety, and behavioral issues like stereotypic behaviors (weaving, cribbing, stall walking). However, effective management of group dynamics is necessary to mitigate potential aggression, resource competition, and bullying. Thoughtful consideration of group compatibility, adequate provision of resources like food and water to reduce competition, and careful monitoring can greatly enhance a horse's welfare in a communal setting.

Health: Preventing, Detecting, and Managing Well-being

Health is fundamental to equine welfare, encompassing the prevention, detection, and management of well-being through proactive care and timely medical intervention. Routine veterinary care—including regular vaccinations, parasite control, dental maintenance, and hoof care—is essential for minimizing the risk of illness or injury. Because horses are prey animals, they frequently mask discomfort or pain until a condition becomes severe; therefore, consistent and thorough assessments are critical for early detection and intervention. Ethical management practices also play a significant role in maintaining equine health, including the avoidance of overly restrictive tack, excessive workloads, or harmful training methods involving unnecessary force. Additionally, responsible decision-making at the end of a horse's life is vital, ensuring horses do not endure unnecessary suffering when their quality of life becomes irreversibly compromised.

Behavioral Interactions: Supporting Natural and Ethical Engagement

The fourth domain, Behavioral Interactions, emphasizes the profound importance of allowing horses to engage fully in natural social behaviors, particularly through meaningful herd interactions. Horses are evolutionarily adapted to thrive within complex social structures; thus, prolonged isolation or inadequate social opportunities can lead to severe psychological stress, anxiety, and the manifestation of stereotypic behaviors such as cribbing, weaving, or stall walking. Ensuring horses have consistent and appropriate access to companions, ideally through direct herd turnout or at least ample opportunities for visual and tactile contact with other horses, is essential for maintaining emotional well-being and psychological health. Equally crucial is the quality of human interactions. Ethical, evidence-based training techniques that foster trust, respect, and clear communication should be favored over coercive or fear-based methods, which can lead to stress-induced disorders and learned helplessness. Conversely, employing training methods that are clear, consistent, and aligned with the horse's neurological and social needs not only enhances learning outcomes but also nurtures the horse's confidence, curiosity, and willingness to engage. Additionally, providing environmental enrichment such as varied terrain and opportunities for exploration further promotes mental stimulation, reduces boredom, and complements the beneficial effects of healthy social integration within the herd.

Mental State: The Key to True Welfare

Perhaps the most transformative element of the Five Domains Model is the final domain: Mental State. This domain synthesizes all preceding factors to evaluate a horse's holistic emotional and psychological well-being. Genuine welfare extends beyond merely preventing harm—it involves actively creating an environment of comfort, safety, and positive engagement. A horse may receive adequate nutrition, healthcare, and shelter yet still suffer from chronic stress, anxiety, or frustration, significantly diminishing its overall welfare. Accurately assessing equine emotional and psychological states requires careful observation of behavioral signs, stress responses, and individual temperament. Effective management and training practices must prioritize reducing stressors and actively providing opportunities for pleasure, relaxation, and social connection. Recognizing and fostering positive emotional states—such as contentment, curiosity, and social bonding—allows caregivers to elevate equine welfare from basic adequacy to genuine thriving.

Conclusion: A Proactive Commitment to Equine Welfare

The Five Domains Model presents a progressive and evidence-based framework for assessing and enhancing equine welfare. Instead of merely preventing suffering, it emphasizes the proactive enrichment of horses' lives. This model shifts traditional welfare standards by giving equal weight to physical health and psychological and emotional experiences. By embedding these principles into routine care, training, and veterinary practices, horse owners and equine professionals can ensure continuous improvement in welfare outcomes. A horse's quality of life should be measured not only by freedom from discomfort and distress but also by the consistent presence of fulfillment, security, and meaningful engagement. Through informed and compassionate practices, we can foster conditions where horses not only survive but genuinely thrive, experiencing full lives characterized by comfort, security, and positive interactions.

Nutrition

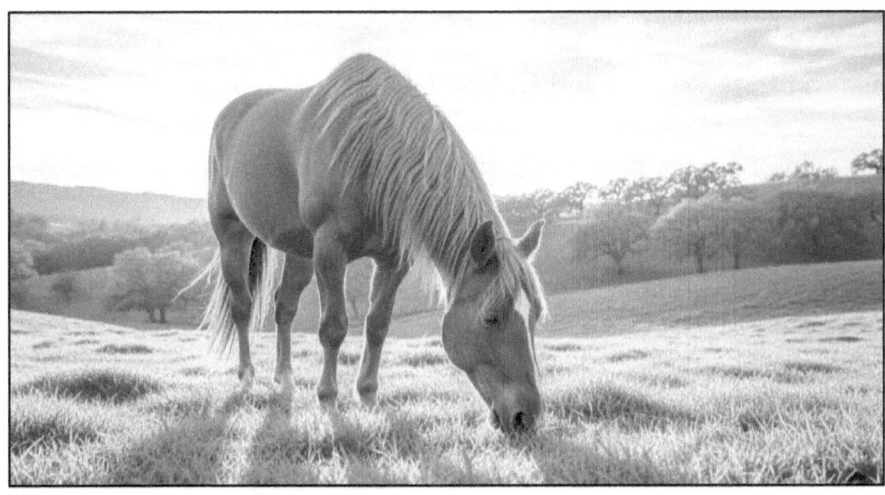

Nutrition is a fundamental pillar of equine welfare, as outlined in the Five Domains Model, directly influencing a horse's physical health, physiological stability, and overall well-being. Adequate and species-appropriate nutrition not only sustains life but also plays a crucial role in preventing disease, supporting optimal body condition, and promoting behavioral health. Horses are natural grazers, evolved to consume a steady intake of forage-rich diets, and disruptions to this natural feeding pattern, such as insufficient fiber, prolonged fasting, or excessive concentrates, can contribute to metabolic disorders, colic, gastric ulcers, and stereotypic behaviors. Proper nutrition is also essential for meeting the horse's energy demands relative to its workload, age, and physiological status, ensuring muscle development, immune function, and recovery from exertion or illness. Beyond its biological necessity, feeding also has significant affective and behavioral consequences, as access to appropriate forage allows horses to engage in natural foraging behaviors, reducing stress and promoting psychological well-being. Thus, evidence-based nutritional management is not merely about providing sustenance but about optimizing both physical and emotional welfare, aligning feeding practices with the horse's evolutionary needs and individual requirements.

Concentrate Feeding and Gastric Ulcers

The link between concentrate feeding and gastric ulcers in horses is well established, stemming largely from deviations from their natural grazing behavior. In the wild, horses graze almost continuously, producing saliva that buffers stomach acid while maintaining a constant gut fill that protects the sensitive stomach lining. This steady intake of forage prevents hydrochloric acid from splashing onto vulnerable areas of the stomach, reducing the risk of ulceration. However, domestic horses are often fed high grain concentrate diets with limited access to forage, creating a feeding pattern that disrupts their natural digestive processes and increases the likelihood of ulcers.

Concentrate feeding promotes sporadic eating, leaving the stomach empty for extended periods. When the stomach lacks forage, acid pools and comes into direct contact with unprotected gastric tissue, leading to irritation and ulcer formation. Although saliva production increases during eating, the type and frequency of feeding play crucial roles in maintaining gastric health. Some horses engage in oral stereotypies such as cribbing, which may be an attempt to generate saliva, but these behaviors do not produce enough to adequately coat and protect the stomach lining. As a result, horses prone to gastric discomfort face an even higher risk of developing ulcers.

To support optimal gastrointestinal health, feeding practices should align with the horse's natural grazing patterns. Providing continuous access to forage ensures consistent gut fill and steady saliva production, both of which are essential for buffering stomach acid and protecting the gastric lining.

Proper nutrition is essential during winter, as increased energy demands require horses to consume more forage. Digesting high-fiber hay generates heat through fermentation in the hindgut, helping to maintain body temperature. While horses can eat snow as a water source, this practice is inefficient and requires additional energy. Providing access to unfrozen water is critical to prevent dehydration.

Physical Environment

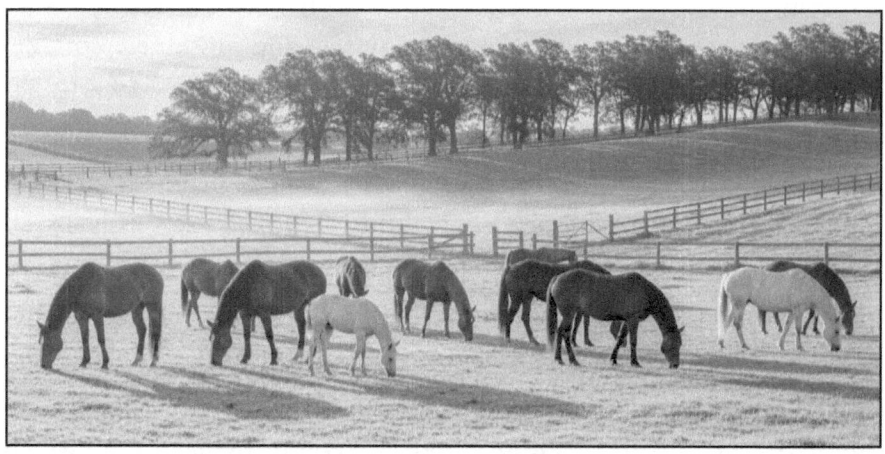

The physical environment plays a foundational role in equine welfare, influencing not just biomechanics but also neurological health, emotional stability, and overall well-being. Movement and space, key components of this domain, are deeply intertwined with the horse's evolutionary adaptations as a cursorial species designed for near-constant locomotion across varied terrain. The neurobiology of movement is closely linked to the mesolimbic reward system, where natural locomotion releases endorphins and promotes dopamine signaling, reinforcing exploratory behaviors and reducing stress. When horses are confined, whether in box stalls, small paddocks, or spaces that lack social and environmental enrichment, their normal sensory and motor processing is disrupted. This can result in heightened stress reactivity, impaired cognitive flexibility, and the emergence of stereotypic behaviors such as weaving and cribbing. Chronic restriction of movement can also maintain the hypothalamic-pituitary-adrenal (HPA) axis in a state of heightened activation, contributing to long-term stress.

Enclosure size and design significantly impact horses' behavioral expression and welfare. Research demonstrates that smaller enclosures correlate with increased frustration and stereotypic behaviors such as pacing and milling. In contrast, larger, enriched environments allow for natural behaviors such as grazing, social bonding, and play, all of which regulate the autonomic nervous system and promote emotional balance. Social isolation further compounds welfare concerns, as sensory and social deprivation have profound neurobiological consequences. Studies show that isolation stunts dendritic growth, limiting neural plasticity and adaptability. Horses raised in isolation often lack critical social skills, leading to maladaptive behaviors and difficulty integrating into group settings. In other species, such as zoo animals, chronic stress from enclosure design led to reproductive and digestive dysfunctions until environmental enrichment was prioritized. Similarly, the "Pasture Paradise" model for equine management, which promotes continuous movement, social interaction, and access to forage has been shown to enhance both physical and mental well-being.

One particularly concerning management practice is the widespread use of solitary confinement in box stalls, which amounts to sensory deprivation. Solitary confinement is recognized as psychological torture in humans, yet it remains the industry standard for managing high-value horses under the misconception that isolation equates to safety. However, research contradicts this assumption, showing that stalled horses exhibit higher rates of gait abnormalities, lower-limb injuries, lameness, and chronic joint and tendon issues compared to those housed in open environments. Furthermore, solitary housing negatively impacts horses' psychological health, leading to increased stress and behavioral pathologies. Social bonds are essential for equine welfare, as mutual grooming, affiliative behaviors, and proximity within groups contribute to reduced stress and increased emotional resilience. Horses are prey animals that rely on herd dynamics for security and social buffering against environmental stressors, making group living a crucial consideration for welfare-oriented management practices.

Environmental factors also influence horses' sensory and physiological health. Excessive time in stables may contribute to visual impairments, including myopia, due to limited exposure to natural light and reduced opportunities for distance focusing. Horses rely on keen distance vision for detecting predators, making access to outdoor environments essential for maintaining ocular health. Additionally, horses are highly adapted to living outdoors in cold conditions. Their thermoregulatory mechanisms including thick winter coats, piloerection, fat reserves, and behavioral strategies such as huddling for warmth allow them to withstand harsh weather. While blanketing is often used, it can interfere with natural temperature regulation and may cause overheating or sweating, which can be counterproductive. Instead, ensuring horses have adequate forage, shelter, and water is typically sufficient to support their well-being in winter conditions.

Ultimately, aligning management practices with the horse's natural ecological and neurological needs by providing ample space, opportunities for movement, social interaction, and an enriched environment supports cognitive engagement, physical resilience, and emotional balance. By shifting away from restrictive housing models and towards welfare-centered environments, we honor the horse's evolutionary blueprint and foster a life that promotes both health and happiness.

Epigenetics in Horses: While horses inherit a genetic blueprint (genotype) from their parents, the expression of those genes into observable traits and behaviors (phenotype) is shaped by interactions with the environment. During gestation, the genetic blueprint primarily guides the initial formation of the brain and other bodily systems. However, gene expression is dynamically regulated throughout a horse's life, influenced by its experiences and environmental conditions. This ongoing regulation enables the horse's brain and body to adapt to the social and physical environments it encounters.

Epigenetic changes in horses occur when environmental stimuli such as stress, nutrition, training methods, or housing conditions affect gene expression without altering the DNA sequence itself. These changes can involve chemical modifications, such as DNA methylation or alterations to histone proteins, which impact how genes are accessed and read by the body.

The study of equine epigenetics explores how behaviors, management practices, and environmental factors can influence gene expression, effectively "switching" genes on or off. For example, chronic stress caused by inadequate socialization or confinement may activate genes associated with heightened stress responses, while positive experiences, like gentle and consistent handling, may enhance the expression of genes linked to trust and learning.

Importantly, while genetic changes are permanent and inherited, many epigenetic changes are reversible. This offers hope for interventions that can improve a horse's well-being and behavior, such as changes in management, training approaches, and environmental enrichment.

In essence, epigenetics highlights the interplay between a horse's genetic foundation and its environment, showing how experiences can shape biological and behavioral outcomes. This understanding reinforces the importance of providing horses with optimal care and environments that promote their physical, mental, and emotional well-being.

Health

The horse's **gut-brain axis and microbiome** play a fundamental role in overall health, influencing digestion, immune function, behavior, cognition, and emotional well-being. The gut-brain axis is a bidirectional communication network that links the gastrointestinal (GI) tract and the brain through neural pathways, particularly the vagus nerve, as well as hormonal and immune signaling. This complex system regulates mood, stress responses, and appetite via hormones and neurotransmitters such as cortisol, serotonin, and ghrelin. With most the horse's immune cells residing in the gut, the GI tract serves as a crucial hub for both inflammatory responses and behavioral regulation. Recent research has strengthened the connection between gut health and neuroendocrine function, underscoring its role in stress resilience, pain perception, and cognitive flexibility.

The equine microbiome consists of a diverse community of bacteria, fungi, protozoa, and viruses, predominantly residing in the hindgut. These microbes ferment fibrous plant material into volatile fatty acids (VFAs), which serve as a primary energy source for horses. Additionally, the microbiome is responsible for synthesizing essential vitamins, such as B vitamins and vitamin K, supporting immune defense, and maintaining gut integrity. A stable and diverse microbiome is key to digestive efficiency and overall health. However, disruptions due to dietary changes, antibiotic use, stress, or illness can lead to dysbiosis, an imbalance in microbial populations. Dysbiosis has been linked to impaired fiber digestion, increased risk of colic, metabolic dysfunction, and conditions such as laminitis.

Recent studies have reinforced the important connection between the gut microbiome and equine behavior. The gut plays a major role in neurotransmitter production, with approximately 90% of the body's serotonin synthesized in the gut, a neurotransmitter that has influence on mood, stress regulation, and cognitive function. Research suggests that stress-induced microbiome alterations may contribute to behavioral issues such as cribbing, weaving, and heightened anxiety. Furthermore, disruptions in gut health have been linked to changes in learning capacity, problem-solving ability, and even trainability. Emerging studies in both humans and animals indicate that gut microbial diversity may impact neurological function through mechanisms involving neuroinflammation and altered neurotransmitter signaling. These findings emphasize the need for a holistic approach to equine management that prioritizes gut health as a foundation for mental and emotional well-being.

Optimizing the gut-brain axis in horses requires careful dietary and management strategies. A forage-first diet is essential, ensuring continuous access to high-quality fiber to support proper fermentation and microbial balance. Stress reduction through consistent routines, appropriate social interactions, and environmental enrichment helps preserve both gut and brain health. The strategic use of probiotics, which introduce beneficial microbes, and prebiotics, which nourish existing beneficial bacteria, can aid in restoring microbial balance following stress, illness, or antibiotic use. Dietary transitions should be gradual, spanning one to two weeks, to allow the microbiome to adapt and prevent dysbiosis. Monitoring early signs of gut imbalances, such as changes in behavior, inconsistent manure quality, or fluctuations in appetite can help prevent more severe health issues before they escalate.

Future research continues to explore innovative ways to harness microbiome science for equine health and performance. With the aid of advanced sequencing technologies, scientists are now able to map the horse's microbial communities with unprecedented detail, identifying specific microbial signatures associated with both health and disease. One promising therapeutic approach under investigation is fecal microbiota transplantation (FMT), a process in which beneficial microbes from a healthy donor's feces are introduced into the gastrointestinal tract of another animal. In human and veterinary medicine, FMT has shown remarkable success in treating conditions such as Clostridium difficile infection and restoring gut flora after antibiotic use. In horses, FMT is being studied to counteract dysbiosis—a disruption of the microbial ecosystem often triggered by illness, stress, or prolonged antibiotic treatment. Researchers are also investigating whether strategically modulating the equine microbiome could bolster stress resilience, enhance trainability, and support cognitive function through the gut-brain axis. As our understanding deepens, managing the microbiome may prove integral not just to physical recovery, but to cultivating emotional balance and behavioral well-being in the horse.

High hay bags pose a significant risk to horses by increasing the inhalation of dust and airborne particles, which can lead to aspiration and respiratory complications. Feeding at ground level aligns with the horse's natural grazing posture, supporting optimal respiratory health. Research indicates that an elevated head position hinders postural drainage of the respiratory tract, raising the risk of respiratory infections. Additionally, eating from elevated hay nets disrupts the function of the mucociliary escalator, a key mechanism for clearing inhaled particles, while dust plumes from hay nets, especially in enclosed spaces, further increase the risk of chronic conditions such as inflammatory airway disease (IAD).

Pain in horses is more than just a physical sensation, it is a complex experience shaped by neurobiology, psychology, and emotion. While nociception, the detection of harmful stimuli by sensory neurons, is the first step in pain perception, the experience of pain extends beyond this basic process. The brain's interpretation of pain is influenced by past experiences, emotional state, and individual variability, meaning that two horses experiencing the same injury may react very differently.

One of the greatest challenges in equine welfare is distinguishing pain-related behaviors from what is often mislabeled as "bad behavior." Horses that resist commands, show aggression, or appear unwilling to work may not be stubborn or defiant but instead attempting to communicate discomfort. Because horses lack verbal expression, they rely on subtle shifts in body language, movement, and facial expressions to signal distress. When these cues are ignored or misinterpreted, it can lead to unnecessary punishment or training corrections, worsening the underlying issue.

Pain, particularly when it is chronic, can have profound psychological and emotional consequences. It activates the hypothalamic-pituitary-adrenal (HPA) axis, leading to elevated cortisol levels and persistent stress. This chronic activation can impair immune function, disrupt social behaviors, and even contribute to learned helplessness, where a horse ceases to respond to stimuli because it perceives its suffering as inescapable. Pain-related stress also affects learning and cognitive processing, making it harder for horses to focus, retain training, or engage positively with handlers.

Because horses are prey animals, they instinctively mask pain to avoid appearing vulnerable. However, careful observation can reveal key behavioral and physiological indicators of discomfort. Subtle facial expressions such as pinched nostrils, furrowed brows, or tension in the lips can be early warning signs. Changes in posture, weight distribution, or reluctance to move forward may also indicate discomfort. Lameness, often dismissed as a mechanical issue, is frequently an indicator of deeper musculoskeletal pain.

Headshaking in horses secondary to trigeminal neuralgia is a distressing, often chronic condition characterized by sudden, repetitive, and sometimes violent movements of the head, frequently accompanied by signs of discomfort such as snorting, rubbing the face, or striking at the muzzle. The underlying mechanism involves dysfunction or hypersensitivity of the trigeminal nerve, particularly the infraorbital branch, which becomes sensitized and fires abnormally, often in response to otherwise innocuous stimuli such as sunlight, wind, or even vibration. This neuropathic pain is thought to mimic trigeminal-mediated facial pain syndromes in humans, such as trigeminal neuralgia or photic sneeze reflex. Affected horses typically exhibit seasonal or environmental triggers, with symptoms often worsening in spring or summer, possibly due to increased light intensity or allergens. Diagnosis is clinical, based on history and exclusion of other causes, though diagnostic nerve blocks can temporarily alleviate symptoms and thus support the diagnosis. Management strategies are challenging and range from environmental modifications and pharmacologic interventions (such as cyproheptadine, carbamazepine, or gabapentin) to more invasive procedures like percutaneous electrical nerve stimulation or infraorbital neurectomy. However, no single treatment is universally effective, and the prognosis varies. From a neuroscience perspective, headshaking associated with trigeminal neuralgia represents a form of central sensitization, where aberrant afferent signaling creates a persistent pain state, emphasizing the importance of considering neuropathic pain pathways in equine behavioral and medical evaluations.

The Overlooked Impact of Dental Health on Equine Well-Being

Dental discomfort is a commonly overlooked but profoundly influential factor in equine behavior, welfare, and performance. Horses are highly sensitive animals, relying on subtle sensory feedback through the mouth, jaw, and tongue not only for effective mastication, but also for communication, balance, and rein acceptance during ridden work. When dental imbalances arise—such as sharp enamel points, hooks, ramps, or asymmetrical wear—they can cause persistent oral pain. This discomfort may be expressed through behaviors often misinterpreted as defiance or poor training: head tossing, bit evasion, bracing against the reins, reluctance to collect, or general irritability under saddle.

From a neurobiological perspective, chronic or intermittent pain in the mouth activates nociceptive pathways and can heighten sympathetic tone, placing the horse in a persistent state of low-level stress or defensiveness. This can interfere with learning, reduce the horse's tolerance to pressure, and contribute to anxiety or shutdown, especially in training environments that rely heavily on rein-based cues. Over time, undiagnosed dental pain can lead to altered head carriage, cervical tension, and compromised postural alignment—affecting not only performance but also the horse's long-term musculoskeletal health.

When behavioral resistance emerges without clear cause, it is essential to rule out physical discomfort—including dental pathology—before assuming a training problem. Addressing oral health through regular, evidence-informed dental evaluation restores comfort and re-establishes the conditions for relaxation, cooperation, and clear communication. In many cases, restoring functional balance in the mouth is a crucial step in rehabilitating trust and improving the horse's willingness to engage—both neurologically and behaviorally. What may appear as a training issue is often a sensory one, rooted in pain that the horse cannot verbalize but consistently shows through its behavior.

LEARNING, TRAINING, AND WELFARE

"To sleep, perchance to dream."
—William Shakespeare, Hamlet (Act 3, Scene 1)

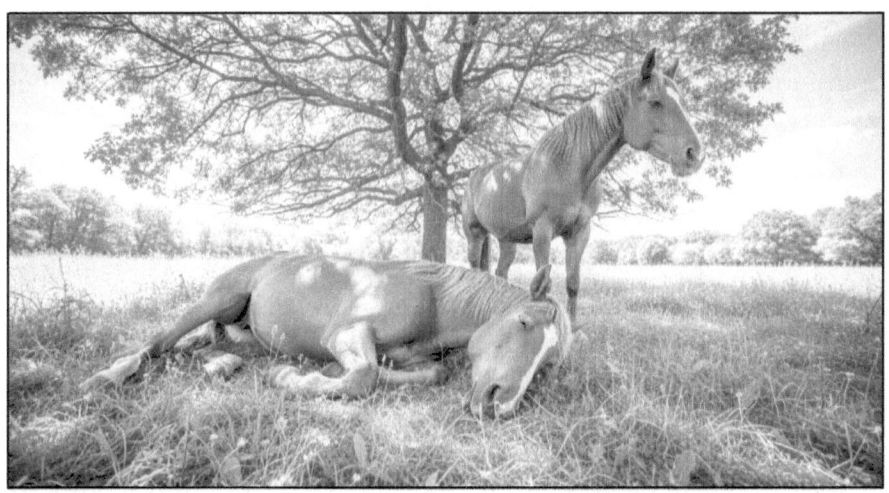

Suprachiasmatic Nucleus and Sleep

The **suprachiasmatic nucleus (SCN),** located within the hypothalamus directly above the optic chiasm, is fundamental in regulating circadian rhythms in mammals, including horses. Receiving direct input from specialized photoreceptive retinal ganglion cells sensitive to blue-wavelength light, the SCN synchronizes internal biological clocks to environmental light-dark cycles. This entrainment orchestrates a variety of physiological processes—such as hormone secretion (including melatonin from the pineal gland), metabolism, and behavioral states—to follow a near 24-hour rhythm, crucial for physiological and behavioral homeostasis.

Horses, like other large mammals, exhibit notably brief sleep durations compared to smaller species, averaging just 3 to 4 hours daily. Despite this limited sleep quantity, its quality and composition remain essential. Neuroscientific research underscores sleep's critical role in cognitive functioning, particularly memory consolidation, a process heavily dependent on mechanisms like long-term potentiation (LTP). During sleep, especially REM (rapid eye movement) sleep, neural circuits involved in recent learning experiences become selectively reactivated, facilitating synaptic strengthening and transitioning memories from short-term storage in the hippocampus to long-term cortical networks. Additionally, sleep serves an indispensable restorative function, allowing cellular repair, metabolic replenishment, and regulation of neuroinflammatory processes.

Horses display unique sleep behaviors and adaptations distinct from many other mammals. Their specialized musculoskeletal structure, termed the stay apparatus, allows horses to remain standing with minimal muscular effort. This anatomical adaptation enables horses to achieve non-REM (NREM) sleep stages while standing, particularly lighter stages of slow-wave sleep (SWS). However, deeper stages of NREM and crucial REM sleep necessitate recumbency, either lying fully on their sides or at least positioning their heads on the ground. This requirement emerges from the characteristic muscle atonia (temporary muscle paralysis) during REM sleep, an evolutionary safeguard preventing acting out vivid dreams or motor behaviors during this neurologically active state.

Given that REM sleep significantly contributes to neural plasticity, synaptic pruning, emotional regulation, and cognitive efficiency, its deprivation carries pronounced consequences. In horses, REM sleep deprivation—commonly due to environmental insecurity, discomfort, or social stress—can induce considerable cognitive impairment, poor decision-making, increased injury risk, and episodic collapse as the brain attempts to enter REM sleep during standing postures. Chronic sleep deprivation, particularly of REM sleep, increases oxidative stress, alters inflammatory cytokine profiles, and diminishes overall physiological resilience.

Numerous factors contribute to insufficient REM sleep in horses. Evolutionarily wired as prey animals, horses possess an innate vigilance and a heightened sensitivity to potential threats, making environmental and psychological security critical prerequisites for comfortable recumbency. Disturbances such as noisy, unsafe stall environments, suboptimal stall design, insufficient or uncomfortable bedding, and stressful herd interactions can all inhibit restful lying-down behaviors. Physical ailments like arthritis, musculoskeletal pain, gastric ulcers, or neurological disorders further compound discomfort, discouraging recumbency. Socially, dominant or aggressive herd mates or sudden changes in herd dynamics can exacerbate chronic sleep insufficiency, underscoring the complex interplay between psychological and physical factors influencing sleep quality.

Equine sleep specialist Dr. Joseph Bertone emphasizes the critical misunderstanding regarding equine sleep patterns—while horses can enter lighter sleep stages standing, essential REM sleep remains impossible without recumbency. Underdiagnosis of sleep deprivation is common, given the subtlety and misinterpretation of its clinical manifestations. Horses suffering chronic sleep deprivation may demonstrate forelimb buckling, frequent stumbling, and episodic collapses to the knees, typically resulting in distinctive scars and abrasions on the dorsal surfaces of fetlocks due to repetitive falls.

An important neurological consequence of prolonged REM deprivation is REM rebound—a compensatory response whereby the brain attempts to recover lost REM sleep. During REM rebound episodes, intensified neuronal firing patterns can provoke pronounced muscle twitching, rapid eye movements, exaggerated limb movements, and, if standing, sudden collapses. Severe REM rebound events may feature thrashing or rhythmic limb movements during recumbency, easily mistaken for seizure-like activities. Horses experiencing these episodes often emit vocalizations—such as snorting or whinnying—which can be distressing to observers unfamiliar with their neurological basis.

Contemporary electroencephalographic (EEG) research reveals striking similarities between the brainwave patterns observed during REM sleep and wakeful states. This neuronal activation pattern, particularly evident in regions associated with memory processing, emotional regulation, and motor planning, underscores REM sleep's pivotal role in maintaining cognitive health and neural adaptability. Consequently, ensuring optimal sleep hygiene and quality is vital in equine management. Practical recommendations include providing secure, quiet resting environments, sufficient comfortable bedding, timely veterinary intervention for painful conditions, and careful attention to herd social structures and interactions to minimize stress-induced vigilance.

Finally, clear distinctions between sleep deprivation and neurological conditions like narcolepsy are critical. Sleep deprivation is primarily caused by modifiable environmental and physiological factors and is reversible through appropriate management. Narcolepsy, on the other hand, involves neurological dysregulation within sleep-wake regulatory circuits and typically necessitates clinical intervention. Understanding these distinctions is crucial to avoid diagnostic errors and to implement targeted interventions effectively.

Behavioral Interactions

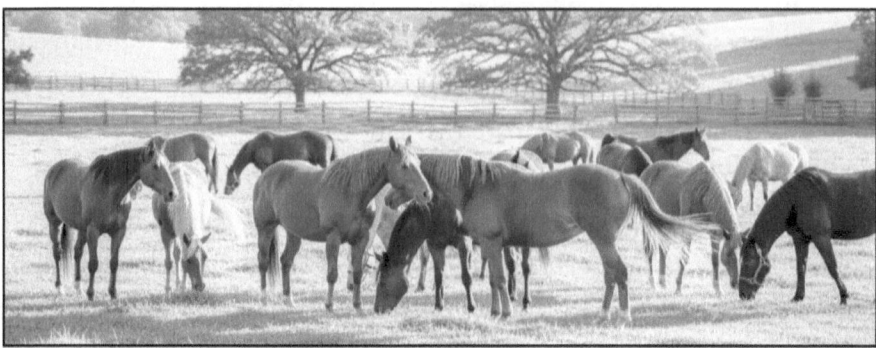

Horses are deeply social creatures, and their neurobiology reflects this intricate social nature. Their brains and neuroendocrine systems are finely tuned for connection, with structures like the amygdala and hippocampus playing key roles in emotional processing and memory, while hormones such as oxytocin and cortisol regulate bonding, stress, and trust. These biological mechanisms underscore the importance of behavioral interactions in equine welfare, influencing herd dynamics, learning, and overall emotional well-being. Recognizing how horses form relationships, both with their peers and with humans, allows us to create environments that foster their social needs rather than work against them.

Scientific research has confirmed what experienced horse people have long observed: horses experience a wide spectrum of emotions, ranging from fear and pain, which are essential for survival, to curiosity and surprise, which facilitate learning and adaptation. These affective states shape their interactions with their environment and with one another. While horses may not process emotions with the same abstract complexity as humans, their behavioral and physiological responses reveal a rich emotional life finely attuned to their evolutionary needs. Recognizing their capacity for attachment and social cohesion deepens our understanding of their behavior and underscores the importance of management practices that support, rather than suppress, these intrinsic needs.

At the heart of equine behavior is trust—a fundamental element that influences every aspect of a horse's interaction with humans. Without trust, survival-driven instincts take precedence, often leading to behaviors misinterpreted as resistance or defiance by those unfamiliar with equine cognition. What may appear as disobedience is frequently a response to fear, discomfort, or confusion. When a horse resists, it is not being willfully defiant but rather communicating that something in its environment is not working. Instead of imposing control, fostering trust requires patience, attunement, and respect for the horse's perception of the world. Every interaction—whether in training, handling, or daily care—shapes the horse's sense of safety and confidence, ultimately influencing the depth and quality of its relationship with humans.

Horses are inherently social and thrive on movement and interaction. In their natural environment, they travel great distances daily, engaging in foraging, play, and social bonding. However, many modern management systems severely restrict these natural behaviors, confining horses to stalls for prolonged periods and limiting their social exposure. Such restrictions can lead to frustration, stress, and the development of stereotypic behaviors like cribbing, weaving, and stall-walking, clear indicators of unmet psychological and physical needs. Equally detrimental is social isolation, which deprives horses of the companionship and mutual support they rely on for emotional stability. Providing opportunities for turnout, socialization, and unrestricted movement is fundamental to their well-being.

The relationship between a human and a horse is a dynamic exchange between two complex cognitive and emotional systems. Each horse possesses a unique neurological makeup shaped by genetics, past experiences, and environmental factors. To engage effectively, we must recognize these individual differences and approach interactions with sensitivity. Fear, confusion, and even curiosity are not signs of defiance but rather attempts to communicate. Punishing a horse for these natural responses only serves to erode trust and stifle authentic interaction. By learning to read subtle cues in the horse's ears, eyes, nostrils, and body tension, we move beyond mechanical responses and into a space of true connection. Only through attentive listening and thoughtful engagement can we cultivate a relationship that is not only effective but also deeply respectful of the horse's intrinsic behavioral needs.

Mental State

The mental state of a horse is a fundamental aspect of its overall welfare and is explicitly recognized within the Five Domains Model of animal welfare. While traditional assessments often focused primarily on physical health and survival needs, modern understandings, particularly those informed by neuroscience, underscore the importance of an animal's emotional and cognitive experiences. A horse's mental state is shaped by its ability to engage with its environment, form social bonds, experience positive interactions and avoid negative emotional states such as fear, stress, and frustration. Neuroscientific research has demonstrated that chronic stress, anxiety, or learned helplessness can lead to profound changes in the equine brain, impairing learning, increasing reactivity, and negatively impacting overall functioning. Prolonged exposure to stressors can dysregulate the hypothalamic-pituitary-adrenal (HPA) axis, leading to maladaptive behavioral responses and diminished cognitive function.

Conversely, a horse that experiences mental security, positive engagement, and a sense of control over its environment is more likely to exhibit curiosity, relaxation, and a willingness to learn. The Five Domains Model moves beyond simply minimizing suffering to actively promoting positive mental states, ensuring that horses can experience comfort, confidence, and even enjoyment in their interactions with humans and their surroundings. The neurobiology of learning and emotion supports this perspective, as positive experiences, clear communication, and predictable environments facilitate the release of neurotransmitters such as, serotonin and dopamine which enhance learning and foster a sense of emotional balance and motivation.

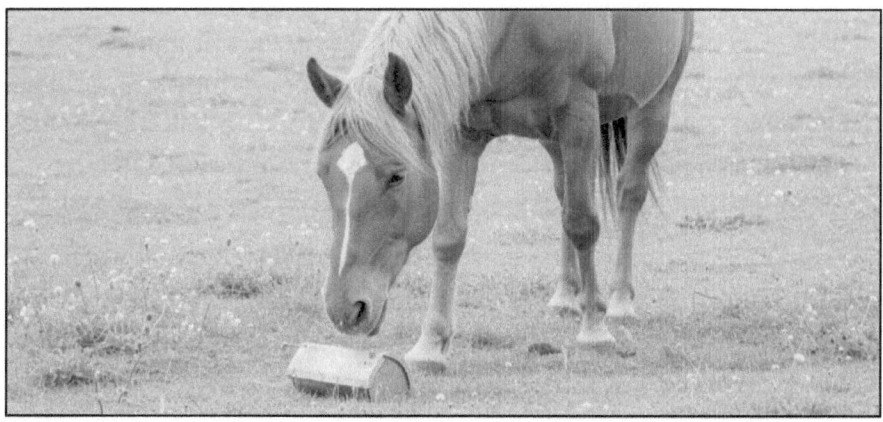

The mental health of the horse must always take precedence over the pursuit of trained behaviors. Ethical training is not merely about achieving desired responses; it is a commitment to methods that respect the horse's cognitive and emotional well-being. A truly ethical approach ensures that learning enhances, rather than compromises, the horse's mental state by aligning with how the equine brain naturally processes information. This means avoiding techniques that induce fear, confusion, or unnecessary stress and instead fostering clarity, trust, and a sense of security. By prioritizing psychological welfare, training becomes not only more effective but also a pathway to a deeper, more humane partnership between horse and handler—one built on mutual understanding rather than coercion.

Behavioral enrichment plays a crucial role in neuroplasticity, the brain's ability to reorganize itself by forming new neural connections throughout life. In the context of equine welfare, enrichment, through social interaction, novel stimuli, problem-solving tasks, and opportunities for natural behaviors, stimulates sensory, motor, and cognitive pathways, reinforcing adaptive learning and resilience. Horses that experience varied and engaging environments exhibit increased synaptic activity and structural changes in brain regions associated with learning, memory, and emotional regulation. Conversely, animals deprived of enrichment may suffer from neural atrophy, heightened stress responses, and maladaptive behaviors due to misbalanced neurochemical engagement. Providing diverse sensory, cognitive, and physical challenges not only enhances equine well-being but also strengthens the neural architecture necessary for flexibility in learning, emotional stability, and overall adaptability. Thus, behavioral enrichment is not merely a welfare consideration; it is a fundamental component of brain health, shaping an equine's ability to respond to its environment with confidence, curiosity, and resilience.

Cognitive Dysfunction Syndrome: Can Horses Develop Dementia?

The question of whether horses can develop dementia has intrigued veterinarians and neuroscientists alike. So far, findings in equine brain pathology have not shown significant evidence of advanced small vessel ischemic changes or cerebrovascular alterations indicative of vascular dementia, a common form of dementia in humans. While there is evidence of beta-amyloid plaques in horse brains, one of the hallmarks of Alzheimer's disease in humans, research has not yet identified the neurofibrillary tangles in areas such as the entorhinal cortex of the hippocampus that are strongly linked to Alzheimer's-related clinical signs. This absence of certain pathological markers makes it difficult to draw parallels between equine cognitive decline and human neurodegenerative diseases.

Despite the limited pathological evidence, horses can exhibit behavioral and cognitive changes that resemble clinical signs of dementia in humans. These signs include alterations in normal habits and personality, a loss of previously learned skills, and disorientation in familiar surroundings. Affected horses may also fail to recognize their owners, display compulsive or repetitive behaviors, and undergo significant changes in eating and drinking habits.

In free-ranging populations, older horses may begin to wander aimlessly, becoming isolated from their herd. Similarly, domestic horses experiencing cognitive decline may withdraw from group activities and, eventually, from the social structure of the herd. Such behavioral changes can reflect a broader dysfunction in cognitive and neurological processes, even if the precise pathological mechanisms remain elusive.

These observations underscore the need for further research into the equine aging brain. Investigating potential links between behavioral symptoms and underlying neuroanatomical or molecular changes could shed light on how aging affects cognition in horses. Additionally, studying equine cognitive dysfunction may offer insights into the evolution of dementia and its manifestation across species, particularly in animals with long lifespans and complex social behaviors like horses.

Stereotypic Behaviors in Horses: A Neuroendocrinological Perspective on Stress and Adaptation

Stereotypies in horses, such as cribbing, weaving, and stall-walking, are often viewed as undesirable behaviors, but from a neuroscientific perspective, they serve as effective adaptive strategies to mitigate stress and regulate cortisol levels. These repetitive behaviors emerge in response to chronic stressors such as social isolation, gastrointestinal discomfort, confinement, or inconsistent training methods that trigger dysregulation of the autonomic nervous system. When a horse engages in a stereotypy, the behavior can activate endogenous reward pathways, particularly those involving the dopaminergic system and lower cortisol levels which provides temporary relief from stress-induced neurochemical imbalances helping the horse regain some degree of physiological homeostasis.

From a neuroendocrinological perspective, stereotypies are deeply rooted in the dysregulation of neurotransmitter systems, particularly those involving dopamine and serotonin. Dopaminergic hypersensitization, particularly in the mesoaccumbens pathway, plays a central role in the development of stereotypic behaviors. Chronic stress leads to elevated baseline levels of beta-endorphins, endogenous opioids that provide pain relief and induce pleasure. This neurochemical shift super sensitizes dopamine neurons within the nucleus accumbens (an area of the brain associated with motivation and reinforcement learning) resulting in a heightened response to self-reinforcing behaviors such as cribbing.

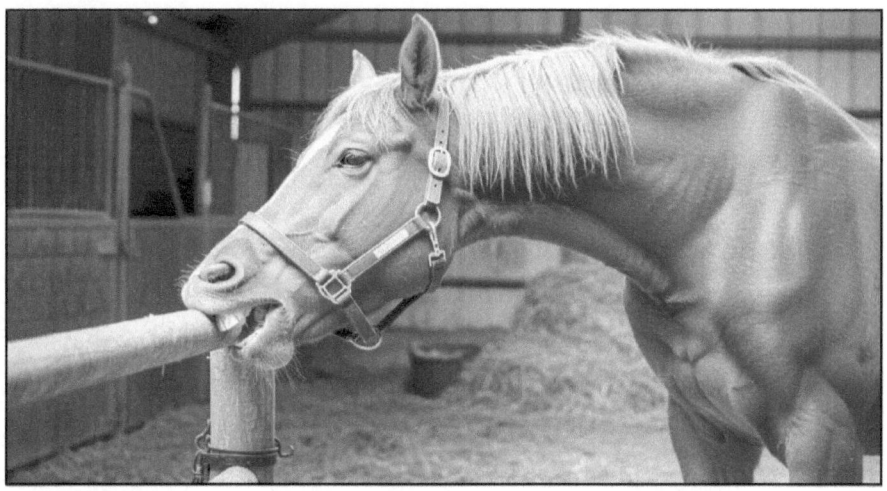

Additionally, research indicates that horses exhibiting stereotypic behaviors have reduced levels of serotonin, a neurotransmitter crucial for emotional regulation and stress mitigation. Decreased serotonergic activity, coupled with increased dopaminergic stimulation, contributes to compulsive behaviors that become ingrained and difficult to eliminate. Over time, stereotypies mimic addictive behaviors, wherein the affected horse experiences a reinforcing dopamine surge each time the behavior is performed, perpetuating a cycle of repetition and dependence.

The mesoaccumbens pathway, a subset of the mesolimbic dopamine system, connects the ventral tegmental area (VTA) to the nucleus accumbens and plays a key role in processing rewards and driving motivated behavior. In environments that fail to meet a horse's intrinsic needs such as prolonged confinement or isolation, dopaminergic dysregulation within this pathway fosters the development of stereotypic behaviors. The repeated performance of cribbing or weaving triggers dopamine release, providing temporary relief from stress but reinforcing the behavior's persistence.

Similarly, the nigrostriatal dopamine system, which connects the substantia nigra to the dorsal striatum, governs motor planning and voluntary movement. Disruptions in this system may contribute to the compulsive, repetitive nature of stereotypies, as horses deprived of appropriate outlets for movement engage in fragmented, self-reinforcing motor patterns. This neurological inflexibility further entrenches stereotypies, making them resistant to behavioral suppression.

Stereotypic behaviors in horses do not emerge randomly; they are the result of exposure to environmental stressors and management practices that fail to align with the species' natural behavioral repertoire. Several key factors contribute to the development and persistence of these behaviors. Restricted foraging is a major factor, as horses are biologically adapted to graze for 16–18 hours per day. Diets high in concentrates and low in fiber disrupt natural feeding rhythms, increasing stress and frustration. Limited social interaction is another significant contributor. As highly social animals, horses rely on herd dynamics for emotional stability, and isolation from conspecifics elevates stress and predisposes horses to stereotypic behaviors. Confinement and restricted movement also play a role, as prolonged stall confinement without sufficient turnout or exercise leads to frustration and heightened stress responses. Abrupt weaning further exacerbates stress in young horses. In natural conditions, foals remain with their mothers for up to two years, and premature weaning disrupts social bonding and contributes to heightened stress levels.

There is no scientific evidence to support the idea that stereotypies are learned through social observation. Instead, their occurrence within a group of horses is more accurately attributed to shared environmental stressors. Research in neuroscience and neuroendocrinology suggests that these behaviors develop as individual coping mechanisms in response to chronic stress. Genetic predisposition also plays a role, as certain breeds, such as Arabians, have a higher density of dopamine neurons and may be more susceptible to dopaminergic dysregulation, making them more prone to developing stereotypic behaviors.

Given that stereotypies serve as coping mechanisms which reduce cortisol levels, efforts to eliminate them through aversive conditioning or physical restraints are neither ethical nor effective. Such interventions often exacerbate stress and negatively impact welfare. Instead, management strategies should focus on mitigating the underlying stressors that drive these behaviors. Enhancing foraging opportunities by providing ad libitum hay or using slow feeders encourages natural grazing behaviors, reducing frustration. Increasing social interaction by allowing horses to engage in group turnout fosters social bonds and reduces stress. Maximizing movement through ample turnout and varied exercise opportunities helps alleviate frustration and maintain mental well-being. Implementing humane weaning practices with gradual strategies reduces stress in young horses, lowering the risk of developing stereotypies. Offering environmental enrichment minimizing boredom and stress.

By addressing the root causes of stress and prioritizing environmental enrichment, social opportunities, and naturalistic management practices, caregivers can significantly reduce the prevalence of stereotypic behaviors.

Anthropomorphism

> "*Go right to the source and ask the horse.*"
> —Mister Ed *(American television sitcom, early 1960s)*

Let Horses Be Horses — Overcoming the Pitfalls of Anthropomorphism

One of the most persistent obstacles to understanding horses clearly and compassionately is anthropomorphism—the human tendency to project our own thoughts, emotions, and intentions onto animals. While emotional connection with horses is deeply meaningful, interpreting equine behavior through a human psychological framework can lead to profound misjudgments, both in training and in care. Horses are not humans in hooved bodies; they are prey animals with evolutionary adaptations and neurobiological processes that differ significantly from our own. Recognizing this difference does not diminish the bond we can share with them—it elevates it. It gives us the tools to relate to horses based not on assumption, but on understanding.

The equine brain has evolved to prioritize safety, sensory vigilance, and rapid motor responses. Behaviors that might appear to reflect humanlike traits—such as determination, stubbornness, defiance, or affection—are more accurately interpreted as outcomes of specific neurophysiological states. For instance, what some might describe as "boldness" in a horse may be the result of elevated norepinephrine levels, creating a heightened state of vigilance that looks like confidence but may be underpinned by anxiety. Similarly, a horse labeled as "lazy" or "difficult" is often expressing confusion, stress, or learned patterns stored in the basal ganglia—regions involved in procedural memory and habit formation. By misattributing intent to behavior, we risk missing the physiological and cognitive reality driving the horse's response.

This misinterpretation is especially dangerous in training contexts. When a horse spooks, hesitates, or fails to respond to a cue, the underlying cause is typically fear, sensory overload, pain, or a failure to understand. Yet the human impulse to assign motive—"He's testing me," or "She's being disrespectful"—often leads to frustration or even punitive handling. Such interpretations impose a moral framework foreign to the equine brain. Horses do not operate from intention or spite; they respond to patterns of reinforcement, perceived threat, and environmental clarity. Their behavior is shaped by neurochemistry, learning history, and the immediate sensory landscape—not by logic or emotion as humans experience it.

Perhaps the most damaging misreading of equine behavior is the mistaken interpretation of freeze responses as calmness or compliance. Tonic immobility—a state in which the nervous system essentially locks down when flight is not possible—is a well-documented defense mechanism in prey animals. In this dissociative state, the horse may appear quiet, obedient, or even relaxed, when in fact it is neurologically overwhelmed. Prolonged exposure to inescapable stressors can lead to learned helplessness, a condition in which the horse stops trying to respond or escape, not because it has learned the task, but because it has given up. Understanding this neurobiological reality is essential to creating ethical training environments and avoiding the perpetuation of trauma under the guise of discipline.

Training horses effectively requires attention to the science of how they learn—not how we think they should behave. Reinforcement, not reasoning, governs the horse's world. A consistent framework of negative reinforcement—removing pressure at the moment of the desired response—and, when appropriate, positive reinforcement—offering something the horse values—forms the backbone of effective training. Horses do not respond to appeals to fairness, guilt, or intention. They respond to timing, clarity, and repetition. Any assumption that a horse "knows better" or is "acting out" reflects a human-centered lens that obscures what's really happening in the brain and body.

This same lens often informs how horses are managed, with well-meaning but physiologically harmful consequences. The concept of iatrogenesis—harm caused by the caregiver's intervention—is just as applicable to equine care as it is in human medicine. Over-blanketing, for example, reflects the human discomfort with cold, not the horse's. Equines are well adapted to cold climates, growing thick winter coats and generating heat internally through fermentation of fiber in the hindgut. Heavy blanketing, particularly in milder weather or with inadequate movement, can lead to overheating, suppression of thermoregulatory functions, and skin issues. The same can be said for overfeeding grain, another expression of anthropomorphic nurturing. While it may feel like a gift, rich carbohydrate-based meals disrupt the horse's digestive physiology, increase the risk of colic and laminitis, and contribute to insulin resistance and obesity—metabolic dysfunctions with long-term consequences.

Other practices, such as excessive confinement, removal of vibrissae (facial whiskers), or cosmetic grooming, reflect human preferences more than equine needs. Confining horses to stalls for extended periods, while often framed as protective, disrupts their natural movement patterns, social interactions, and gastrointestinal health. The equine body is designed for continuous, low-intensity motion; the mind is wired for sensory input, environmental engagement, and herd communication.

Stabling practices that isolate horses from their peers not only induce boredom and restlessness but also interfere with the horse's primary source of safety: social buffering. Horses kept indoors to avoid mud, or cosmetic mess may be spared minor inconveniences, but often at the cost of psychological and physiological wellbeing.

Even seemingly affectionate gestures—such as constant soothing, petting, or offering treats without structure—can create insecurity or neurochemical dysregulation. Horses thrive on consistency and structure. Their neuroendocrine systems are tuned to predictability. Without clear patterns of reinforcement, well-meaning interactions can become confusing or even provoke food-seeking behaviors that escalate into aggression or anxiety. Overindulgence, framed as kindness, may in fact create dependency or instability.

From a neuroscience perspective, psychological robustness comes not from overprotection, but from exposure to manageable challenges and the opportunity to recover. Resilience develops when a horse is allowed to enter mild sympathetic arousal—engaging the brain's attention and learning circuits—and then return to parasympathetic rest. This adaptive cycling supports autonomic flexibility and confidence. Over-sheltering a horse, or avoiding all discomfort, narrows its experiential window and makes it less capable of regulating itself under stress. The goal is not to eliminate challenge, but to provide it in a context that allows the horse to succeed—and to recover.

In the training arena, anthropomorphism can also dull our observational acuity. Effective horsemanship begins with accurate interpretation. Recognizing tension in the nostrils, bracing in the lumbar spine, pinning of the ears, or subtle shifts in gait requires a neutral lens—not one colored by what we think the horse "feels." The language of the horse is sensory and behavioral, not conceptual. To see clearly, we must observe without projecting. Fluency in equine body language, facial expression, and movement is not just a skill—it is an ethical imperative.

Letting horses be horses means recognizing their needs as distinct from our own and building systems around those needs. It means feeding forage throughout the day to support gastrointestinal function and behavior. It means providing herd interaction, turnout space, appropriate novelty, and a social life that resembles what their nervous systems evolved to expect.

This is not a call for emotional detachment. On the contrary, the more we understand the horse's true nature, the deeper our relationship can become. When we remove the filter of anthropomorphism, we begin to see horses as they are—not as extensions of ourselves, but as intelligent, sensitive, and evolutionarily distinct beings. Respect grows. Communication improves. And care becomes not an act of projection, but of presence.

The neuroscience of the horse calls us to humility. It challenges us to set aside our assumptions and to meet the horse where it lives—through movement, sensation, social context, and survival-based learning. When we replace anthropomorphism with knowledge, we don't lose magic—we gain trust. We honor the horse by listening, adapting, and acting with clarity. To let a horse be a horse is not to love it less, but more—on its own terms, in its own language, and with the full respect its nature deserves.

SECTION IV

Horsemanship Principles

The Principles of an Evidence-Based Approach to Horsemanship

Rethinking the Foundation

Modern horsemanship is undergoing a critical transformation—one driven not by tradition or charisma, but by scientific understanding. This shift moves us from the realm of opinion and anecdote into a framework built on the brain, the body, and how learning truly works. An evidence-based approach emphasizes alignment with the horse's nervous system, endocrine responses, and evolutionary behaviors. It prioritizes not just what "works," but what is repeatable, explainable, and humane.

A horse is not a machine to be programmed or a vessel to be dominated. It is a sentient, learning organism whose brain is constantly reshaping itself based on experience. When training aligns with the underlying neurobiology, learning becomes more efficient, stress is reduced, and the relationship between horse and human deepens. This approach offers clarity in a landscape too often clouded by outdated customs, quick-fix methods, and pseudoscientific claims. Instead of relying on tradition alone, we now have the tools—and the responsibility—to do better.

Learning and the Adaptable Brain

At the heart of any training interaction is neuroplasticity—the horse's capacity to change neural connections in response to experience. Repetition strengthens these connections, particularly in regions such as the sensory and motor cortices, the cerebellum, and the basal ganglia. The basal ganglia are especially important in establishing habits. Once a response becomes patterned and automatic, it shifts from conscious learning to procedural memory. That's why consistent cues and timing matter. Repetition builds reliability. Inconsistency builds confusion.

For a behavior to be learned and retained, it must be rewarded in a timely and meaningful way. Neuroscientific research shows that there's a critical window—often just a few seconds—within which the brain links an action to its outcome. When reinforcement is delayed, or when the horse is unsure which behavior prompted the release of pressure or the delivery of reward, learning degrades. This is not a matter of opinion—it is the physiology of synaptic efficiency.

An evidence-based approach therefore insists on impeccable timing and clarity. It avoids ambiguity in cues, reinforces the desired behavior immediately, and repeats the process often enough to encode the behavior into long-term memory. Training becomes a process of shaping the brain, one repetition at a time.

Hormones, Motivation, and Emotional Safety

Every training interaction takes place within the horse's internal neurochemical environment. Understanding that environment adds depth and precision to our work. Dopamine, for instance, is not just a "feel good" molecule—it signals prediction and reward. It helps reinforce correct responses and supports motivation. When a horse finds relief from pressure or achieves clarity in a task, dopamine helps mark that success, reinforcing neural pathways and encouraging future engagement.

Cortisol, by contrast, is a hormone associated with the stress response. Short-term spikes in cortisol can be adaptive, preparing the body for focused effort. But chronic elevation—especially when caused by unpredictable or aversive handling—leads to dysregulation, poor learning, and long-term welfare concerns. Horses living or training under constant stress are not learning effectively; they are simply surviving.

Oxytocin, associated with bonding and feelings of safety, is released in contexts of trust, familiarity, and gentle touch. It fosters social cohesion and emotional regulation. Norepinephrine modulates arousal and attention—necessary for learning but harmful when pushed into hypervigilance. Serotonin contributes to mood regulation, confidence, and emotional balance, and is influenced by both environment and early social experiences.

To create the best possible learning state, a trainer must minimize unnecessary stress while maintaining attentiveness. This means designing environments that support safety, predictability, and co-regulation between horse and human. Neuroendocrinology reminds us: when the horse feels safe, the brain becomes more plastic. Learning accelerates. Communication improves.

Conditioning, Contingency, and Communication

Effective training is built on principles of operant and classical conditioning, both of which are supported by decades of behavioral science and neuroscience.

Operant conditioning—learning through consequences—guides most training systems. Horses learn through the association between their actions and the resulting outcomes. An evidence-based approach favors negative reinforcement (removal of pressure when the desired response occurs) and positive reinforcement (addition of something the horse finds rewarding, such as food or rest) because these methods support clarity and motivation.

Positive punishment—the addition of an aversive stimulus to stop a behavior—carries significant risks. It can create fear, inhibit learning, and damage trust. Similarly, negative punishment—the removal of something valued—may work in theory but is often misapplied or poorly understood.

Classical conditioning is equally important. It's how a horse learns to associate a sound, cue, or environment with an outcome. For example, a clicker or voice cue can be paired with a food reward, or a specific gesture can come to signal safety. These associations influence how the horse perceives and anticipates the world.

Critically, all forms of conditioning require contingency and consistency. The horse must understand what causes what. Ambiguous cues, mixed signals, or inconsistent application of pressure confuse the horse's nervous system. The result is learned helplessness, anxiety, or resistance—each of which is not a sign of "disobedience" but of an overwhelmed or underinformed brain.

Arousal, Regulation, and the Nervous System

Training does not occur in a vacuum—it is filtered through the horse's autonomic nervous system. Emotional state, sensory input, and physiological arousal all shape how a horse receives and processes information. While much attention is given to the calming influence of the parasympathetic system—the branch responsible for rest, digestion, and recovery—it's important to understand that learning doesn't primarily occur in that mode. Instead, effective learning requires activation of the sympathetic nervous system to a manageable degree. This branch of the nervous system supports attention, engagement, and motor readiness. It is what allows the horse to become alert, responsive, and capable of absorbing new information.

That said, not all sympathetic arousal is beneficial. When arousal escalates into hyperreactivity—when the horse is startled, overwhelmed, or panicked—the capacity for learning diminishes dramatically. At that point, behavior is governed more by reflex and fear than by conscious processing or memory formation. The goal is not to avoid sympathetic activation, but to work within an optimal zone of arousal—what some call the "learning zone" or the zone of proximal development—where challenge is present, but tolerable.

Contrary to the common misconception that learning should always take place in a low-stress comfort zone, meaningful nervous system adaptation often requires moving slightly beyond that zone. When horses are gradually exposed to unfamiliar or mildly challenging stimuli and then allowed to return to a regulated state, their nervous systems build tolerance, flexibility, and resilience. This process—stress exposure followed by recovery—supports the kind of neuroplastic changes that lead to stronger learning and emotional regulation.

An evidence-based approach therefore favors controlled exposure: taking the horse just far enough into sympathetic activation to engage learning systems and then providing the conditions for recovery. This cycle of mobilization and reset creates adaptive capacity. It is how horses develop confidence in the face of novelty, and how they learn to regulate their own nervous systems in partnership with the human. A horse that has never been allowed to experience mild discomfort in a structured, supportive context may be more fragile, not less. The goal is not to avoid all stress, but to build stress tolerance through skillful guidance and clear, repeatable communication.

Ultimately, both arousal and recovery are necessary. Arousal mobilizes attention and energy for learning. Recovery consolidates that learning and restores emotional balance. When used ethically and with awareness of the horse's thresholds, this dynamic dance between sympathetic challenge and parasympathetic recovery becomes one of the most powerful tools in horsemanship.

Ethics, Empathy, and Neurobiological Respect

The application of neuroscience to horsemanship is not only a matter of technique—it is a matter of ethics. To train with an understanding of the horse's brain is to honor the sentience, vulnerability, and adaptability of that brain. An evidence-based approach does not excuse harsh methods under the banner of results. It challenges us to do better.

This approach does not anthropomorphize horses, but neither does it reduce them to unfeeling automatons. It recognizes that their affective states, social needs, and sensory experiences are central to welfare. It teaches us to recognize when behavior is driven by fear, when conflict signals confusion, and when shutdown is mistaken for compliance.

Ethical horsemanship respects that trust is not a shortcut—it is an outcome of clarity, consistency, and emotional safety. And as neuroscience continues to evolve, it will offer increasingly precise ways of assessing pain, stress, cognitive load, and even preference. Our obligation is to listen—and to adapt.

The Path Forward

An evidence-based approach invites constant refinement. It welcomes new data, values feedback from both the horse and the scientific community and remains flexible as knowledge evolves. No single tradition or school of thought holds all the answers. The brain is complex. Behavior is contextual. Science is ongoing.

But what remains constant is this: when we align our methods with the biology of the horse, we reduce suffering and increase understanding. We communicate more clearly. We achieve more with less force. And we build partnerships that are not only functional but fulfilling for both horse and human.

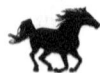

Bridging Science and Practice for the Future

Toward a Scientifically Informed Future of Horsemanship

The future of horsemanship rests not in rigid adherence to tradition, but in our capacity to evolve. As new technologies and scientific insights illuminate the inner workings of the equine brain and body, we find ourselves at a pivotal moment—one where the knowledge to improve welfare, deepen trust, and refine training is within reach, but only if we commit to a more informed, collaborative path. Horsemanship has long been rooted in observation and intuition, but today's landscape calls for more: a blend of lived experience and empirical evidence, grounded in neuroscience, ethology, and behavioral science. At this intersection, the nervous system becomes our guide. It governs perception, movement, emotion, and learning—revealing how horses interpret their world and how we, in turn, must interpret their responses.

Scientific literacy is no longer optional in a world saturated with both valuable information and dangerous misinformation. As horse owners, trainers, and veterinarians face an influx of content online, critical thinking becomes a vital safeguard. Misinformation—unintentional error—can spread as easily as disinformation, which is deliberately deceptive. Both are exacerbated by pseudoscientific claims that may sound impressive but lack peer-reviewed validation. In equestrian settings, such claims might misuse neuroscience terms—like falsely categorizing a horse as "left-brained" or exaggerating the roles of neurotransmitters like dopamine or oxytocin without context. These simplifications distort science and lead to ineffective or even harmful training practices. Understanding the distinctions between sound evidence and seductive jargon is a cornerstone of ethical horsemanship. In an age of viral ideas and influencer authority, intellectual humility, healthy skepticism, and a commitment to lifelong learning are essential traits for the modern equestrian.

Our approach to training must evolve alongside our understanding of equine cognition and neuroplasticity. Behaviors once interpreted as disobedience are increasingly recognized as signs of confusion, stress, or discomfort—often rooted in the horse's limbic system and expressed through hormonal markers like elevated cortisol. This shift toward interpretation over correction fosters clearer communication and a stronger horse-human bond. Future training models will prioritize emotional attunement, positive reinforcement, and environmental predictability, all of which enhance learning and resilience by aligning with how the equine brain processes safety and reward.

The built environment will reflect these neurobiological insights as well. Management practices are moving away from confinement and isolation, toward socially enriched, movement-friendly designs that honor the horse's evolutionary needs. Naturalistic environments such as those modeled after the "Paddock Paradise" concept reduce stress behaviors and improve overall well-being. Early-life socialization—allowing foals to learn from their herds rather than premature human imprinting—builds emotional adaptability and social intelligence, crucial elements for a horse's long-term welfare and trainability. As we refine our understanding of the hippocampus, amygdala, and frontal systems in equine development, we see clearly that psychological safety isn't a luxury—it's a biological necessity.

Emerging technologies now offer tools to further bridge the gap between subjective observation and objective insight. Wearable biometric sensors and AI-assisted monitoring platforms are providing real-time feedback on heart rate variability, locomotion patterns, thermal stress, and more—offering early indicators of pain, fatigue, or emotional distress before clinical signs emerge. The promise of neuroimaging, long limited by the challenges of scale and stress-free data collection, is beginning to take shape through advances in portable, non-invasive tools like EEG and functional near-infrared spectroscopy (fNIRS). These technologies allow us to observe brain activity in real-world settings, giving us clues to how horses process cues, assess risk, and learn through reinforcement. With further refinement, these approaches may help identify early signs of maladaptive plasticity or stress-linked neural changes, giving trainers and caretakers a proactive lens into the horse's inner life.

Longer-term, neuroimaging techniques such as diffusion tensor imaging (DTI) and voxel-based morphometry (VBM) could offer even deeper insight into structural brain differences linked to temperament, cognitive flexibility, or trauma. Though logistical and ethical hurdles remain, the goal is clear: to make equine neuroscience actionable in daily practice. When combined with data from behavioral tracking systems, AI analysis, and endocrinological measures, we are inching closer to a holistic understanding of equine mental and physical states.

This future is not built by scientists alone. It will require collaboration across domains—neuroscientists working with horsemen, ethologists partnering with veterinarians, technologists collaborating with welfare experts. The most effective and ethical horsemanship arises not from one discipline but from an integrated framework. Neuroscience explains nervous systems and brain plasticity; ethology ensures alignment with natural behaviors; learning theory provides consistent, replicable strategies; and equitation science grounds it all in practical, humane application. Together, these disciplines form a triad strengthened by neuroendocrinological insight into the roles of oxytocin, dopamine, serotonin, acetylcholine, and cortisol. This integrated approach supports not only better welfare, but better results—in sport, therapy, recreation, and relationship.

As public scrutiny of equestrian practices increases, the importance of ethical transparency will only grow. The social license to operate depends not on tradition, but on demonstrated commitment to welfare. Regulatory bodies, sponsors, and audiences alike are calling for science-based practices that prioritize the horse's physical and emotional needs. Institutions that lead with integrity—incorporating neuroscience into welfare standards and training systems—will be the ones that endure and influence the next generation.

And it is the next generation—of horses, of humans, of ideas—that holds the greatest promise. The science of neuroplasticity reminds us that change is always possible, at every stage of life. Horses can recover, adapt, and flourish when given the right environment and guidance. So too can humans. As AI continues to evolve, it will serve not as a replacement for horsemen or scientists, but as a tool to accelerate learning, analyze patterns, and distribute knowledge across borders and disciplines. Already, intelligent systems are helping equine researchers mine vast datasets, identify behavioral trends, and develop diagnostic tools. In the future, AI could play a pivotal role in customizing training plans based on biometric feedback, detecting early signs of stress or injury, and supporting ongoing education for equine professionals around the world.

In conclusion, the future of horsemanship is not a rejection of tradition, but a refinement of it through the lens of science, ethics, and empathy. When we learn to see the horse's brain not as a mystery but as a map—one shaped by biology, behavior, and experience—we unlock the potential for deeper connection and more humane, effective practice. Evidence-based horsemanship is not merely a method; it is a mindset—one that values curiosity over certainty, collaboration over dogma, and compassion over control. In honoring the horse's neurobiology, we are called to elevate our own. The more we understand their brain, the more we are asked to refine our own minds, choices, and commitments. In doing so, we don't just shape better horses—we shape a better future.

To those who sensed something deeper behind the science—thank you.

This book explores the equine brain, but beneath the facts runs a quieter rhythm—of nervous systems attuning, of trust becoming biology, of relationship as the root of learning.
If you felt it, you already know:
This isn't just about horsemanship.
It's about returning—
to coherence, to clarity, to the language that lives beneath words.
The signal is always there.
Sometimes, it just takes a horse to help us feel it again.

"If you don't believe me, go ask your horse."
—Dr. Stephen Peters

"The Listening Brain"
by Dr. Stephen Peters

We live in a world where sound never stops.
Yet the art of listening remains profoundly rare.

The horse—a creature of prey—
listens not just with its ears,
but with its nervous system.
It listens for safety, for subtlety, for sincerity.

And what about us?

The human brain—
complex, pattern-seeking, ever-adaptive—
filters signal from noise with astonishing precision.

Attention, guided by *acetylcholine*, sharpens our focus.
Emotion, balanced by *serotonin*, steadies our lens.
Motivation, driven by *dopamine*, fuels our curiosity.

These are not abstractions.
They are the neurochemical symphony behind every moment of understanding.

And in the quiet space between words—
that is where true connection begins.
Not with dominance. Not with force.
But with presence. With patience. With trust.

In the end, the brain learns best—
not under threat,
but through clarity.

And yet—
under the right conditions,
with safety, trust, and repetition,
both horses and humans
can learn to find coherence,
even in the midst of chaos.

GLOSSARY OF KEY TERMS

A

Acetylcholine – A neurotransmitter involved in attention, learning, and muscle activation, playing a crucial role in motor control and memory

Action Potential – A rapid electrical signal that travels along a neuron's axon, enabling communication between neurons.

Adrenal Glands – Small glands above the kidneys that release hormones like cortisol and adrenaline in response to stress.

Afferent Neurons – Sensory neurons that carry information from the body to the central nervous system.

Allostasis – The process by which an organism maintains stability through physiological and behavioral change, often in response to stress.

Amygdala – A brain region crucial for processing emotions, especially fear and threat perception in horses.

Anterior Pituitary (Adenohypophysis) – The front portion of the pituitary gland that secretes hormones such as ACTH, FSH, LH, GH, and TSH, regulating growth, metabolism, and reproductive functions.

Associative Learning – A learning process in which a horse links two stimuli together, such as in classical or operant conditioning.

Autonomic Nervous System (ANS) – The part of the nervous system that controls involuntary functions, such as heart rate and digestion, divided into the sympathetic (fight-or-flight) and parasympathetic (rest-and-digest) systems.

Axon – The long, slender projection of a neuron that conducts electrical impulses (action potentials) away from the cell body toward other neurons or target cells.

B

Basal Ganglia – Brain structures involved in motor control, habit formation, and procedural learning in horses.

Blood-Brain Barrier (BBB) – A selective physiological barrier formed by specialized endothelial cells that restricts the passage of substances from the bloodstream into the brain, maintaining a stable environment for neuronal function.

Brainstem – The lower part of the brain responsible for vital functions such as breathing, heart rate, and arousal.

C

Cerebellum – The brain structure responsible for coordination, balance, and motor learning in horses.

Cerebral Aqueduct – A channel connecting the third and fourth ventricles, containing cerebrospinal fluid.

Cerebral Cortex – The outer layer of the brain involved in higher cognitive functions such as decision-making and sensory processing.

Cerebrospinal Fluid (CSF) – A clear fluid produced by the choroid plexus that circulates within the brain's ventricles and spinal canal, providing cushioning, nutrient delivery, and waste removal.

Classical Conditioning – A learning process where a horse associates a neutral stimulus with a meaningful event (e.g., Pavlovian conditioning).

Corpus Callosum – A large band of nervous tissue that connects the two cerebral hemispheres.

Cortisol – A hormone released in response to stress, influencing energy metabolism and immune function.

Cranial Nerves – Twelve pairs of nerves that emerge directly from the brain and brainstem, controlling functions like facial sensation, eye movements, balance, hearing, and taste.

D

Dendrites – Branch-like structures of neurons that receive signals from other neurons.

Dopamine – A neurotransmitter involved in reward, motivation, and movement, playing a key role in reinforcement learning in horses.

E

Endocrine System – A system of glands that release hormones regulating mood, growth, and behavior.

Endorphins – Endorphins are "endogenous morphine like" *chemicals or hormones that your body releases when it feels pain or stress.*

Equine Ethology – The study of natural horse behavior in relation to neuroscience and training.

Executive Function – Cognitive processes such as problem-solving, impulse control, and working memory.

F

Fear Conditioning – A type of associative learning where a horse learns to associate a stimulus with fear, often leading to long-term behavioral responses.

Frontal Cortex – The area of the brain involved in decision-making, attention and voluntary motor movement though less developed in horses than in humans.

G

GABA (Gamma-Aminobutyric Acid) – The primary inhibitory neurotransmitter in the brain, helping regulate relaxation and reducing excitability.

Glial Cells – Supportive cells in the nervous system that maintain neuron function, including myelin production and immune response.

Glutamate – The primary excitatory neurotransmitter involved in learning and memory.

Gray Matter – The part of the brain consisting mainly of neuronal cell bodies, responsible for processing information.

H

Herd Dynamics – The social structure and interactions within a group of horses, including leadership, dominance, and cooperative behaviors.

Hippocampus – A brain structure essential for learning, memory, and spatial navigation in horses.

Homeostasis – The body's ability to maintain stable internal conditions, regulated by the nervous and endocrine systems.

Hormones – Chemical messengers that travel through the bloodstream to regulate behavior and physiological functions.

HPA Axis (Hypothalamic-Pituitary-Adrenal Axis) – A system of interactions between the hypothalamus, pituitary gland, and adrenal glands that regulates stress responses, mood, and energy.

Hypothalamus – A critical region in the forebrain that regulates autonomic functions like appetite, thirst, body temperature, and circadian rhythms.

I

Inhibitory Control – The ability to suppress impulsive reactions, crucial for training horses to respond to cues.

Interneurons – Neurons that communicate between sensory and motor neurons within the central nervous system.

L

Limbic System – The brain network involved in emotions, motivation, and learning, including the amygdala, hippocampus, and hypothalamus.

Lobes of the Brain – The cerebrum is divided into four main lobes; each associated with different functions:

- **Frontal Lobe:** Associated with attention, decision-making, problem-solving, and voluntary movement.
- **Parietal Lobe:** Processes sensory information related to touch, proprioception, and spatial awareness.
- **Temporal Lobe:** Important for auditory processing, memory, and emotional regulation.
- **Occipital Lobe:** Primarily responsible for visual processing.

Long-Term Potentiation (LTP) – A process that strengthens synaptic connections, crucial for learning and memory formation.

M

Memory Consolidation – The process of stabilizing a memory after initial acquisition, often occurring during sleep.

Motor Cortex – The part of the brain responsible for voluntary movement.

Myelin – A fatty substance that insulates nerve fibers, speeding up neural communication.

N

Negative Reinforcement – The removal of an aversive stimulus to strengthen a desired behavior in training.

Neocortex – The part of the brain involved in higher-order functions like perception and cognition, though less developed in horses.

Neuroendocrinology – The study of the interactions between the nervous system and the endocrine system.

Neurogenesis – The process of new neuron formation in the brain.

Neuroplasticity – The brain's ability to reorganize itself by forming new neural connections, essential for learning.

Neurotransmitters – Chemical messengers that transmit signals between neurons. Examples: Acetylcholine, Dopamine, Serotonin

Norepinephrine – A neurotransmitter and hormone involved in arousal, attention, and the stress response, crucial for alertness and focus.

O

Operant Conditioning – A learning process in which behavior is shaped by reinforcement or punishment.

Oxytocin – A hormone linked to social bonding, trust, and relaxation in horses.

P

Parasympathetic Nervous System – The division of the ANS that promotes relaxation and digestion.

Proprioception – The horse's ability to sense its body position and movement.

R

Reinforcement – A consequence that increases the likelihood of a behavior occurring again.

T

Thalamus – A brain structure that relays sensory information to the cerebral cortex.

Threshold – The level of stimulation required to trigger a neural response or behavioral reaction.

W

Welfare – The overall physical and mental well-being of horses, influenced by training methods, management, and environmental conditions.

BIBLIOGRAPHY

Aleman, M., Williams, D. C., Holliday, T. A., Fletcher, D. J., & Madigan, J. E. (2014). Sensory evoked potentials of the trigeminal nerve for the diagnosis of idiopathic headshaking in a horse. *Journal of Veterinary Internal Medicine, 28*(1), 250–253.

Alves, M., & Bueno, O. (2017). Retroactive interference: Forgetting as an interruption of memory consolidation. *Trends in Psychology, 25*(3), 195–210.

Ambrojo, K. S., Yenisetti, S. C. (Ed.). (2018). Physiology and metabolic anomalies of dopamine in horses: A review. In *Dopamine – Health and Disease*. IntechOpen.

Appleton, J. (2018). The gut-brain axis: Influence of microbiota on mood and mental health. *Integrative Medicine: A Clinician's Journal, 17*(4), 28–32.

Arencibia, A., Rivero, M. A., Gil, F., Vázquez, J. M., Ramirez, J. A., & González, M. (2005). Magnetic resonance imaging of the normal equine brain. *Veterinary Radiology & Ultrasound, 46*(3), 215–222.

Azmitia, E. C. (1999). Serotonin neurons, neuroplasticity, and homeostasis of neural tissue. *Neuropsychopharmacology, 21*(2), 33–45.

Bachmann, I., Bernasconi, P., Herrmann, R., Weishaupt, M. A., & Stauffacher, M. (2003). Behavioural and physiological responses to an acute stressor in crib-biting and control horses. *Applied Animal Behaviour Science, 82*(4), 297–311.

Bachmann, I., Stauffacher, M., Bernasconi, P., & Weishaupt, M. A. (2013). Risk factors associated with behavioural disorders of crib-biting, weaving and box-walking in Swiss horses. *Equine Veterinary Journal, 35*(2), 158–163.

Bacon, S. J., Headlam, A. J., & Gabbott, P. L. (1996). Amygdala input to medial prefrontal cortex in the rat: A light and electron microscope study. *Brain Research, 720*(1–2), 211–219.

Baragli, P., Scopa, C., Maglieri, V., & Sighieri, C. (2021). Horses show individual level lateralization when inspecting an unfamiliar and unexpected stimulus. *PLOS ONE, 16*(8), e0255739.

Baribeau, D. A., & Anagnostou, E. (2015). Oxytocin and vasopressin: Linking pituitary neuropeptides and their receptors to social neurocircuits. *Frontiers in Neuroscience, 9*, 335.

Baxi, K. N., Dorries, K. M., & Wysocki, C. J. (2006). Is the vomeronasal system really specialized for detecting pheromones? *Trends in Neurosciences, 29*(1), 1–7.

Bell, R. J., Kingston, J. K., Mogg, T. D., & Perkins, N. R. (2007). Equine gastric ulcer syndrome in adult horses: A review. *New Zealand Veterinary Journal, 55*(1), 1–12.

Bicego, K. C., Barros, R. C. H., & Branco, L. G. S. (2007). Physiology of temperature regulation: Comparative aspects. *Comparative Biochemistry and Physiology Part A: Molecular & Integrative Physiology, 147*(3), 616–639.

Blake, A. (2015). *Stable Relation: A Memoir of Horses, Healing and Country Living*. Prairie Moon Press.

Blackmore, T. L., Foster, T. M., Sumpter, C. E., & Temple, W. (2008). An investigation of colour discrimination with Equus caballus. *Behavioural Processes, 78*(3), 387–396.

Boissy, A., Manteuffel, G., Jensen, M. B., Moe, R. O., Spruijt, B., Keeling, L. J., Winckler, C., Forkman, B., Dimitrov, I., Langbein, J., Bakken, M., Veissier, I., & Aubert, A. (2007). Assessment of positive emotions in animals to improve their welfare. *Physiology & Behavior*, *92*(3), 375–397.

Boucher, S., Dewulf, L., Henninger, W., & De Lahunta, A. (2020). Diffusion tensor imaging tractography of white matter tracts in the equine brain. *Frontiers in Veterinary Science*, *7*, 382.

Boukhris, O., Boukhris, M., Trabelsi, K., Ammar, A., Masmoudi, L., Souissi, N., & Bragazzi, N. L. (2024). The acute effects of nonsleep deep rest on perceptual responses, physical and cognitive performance in physically active participants. *Applied Psychology: Health and Well-Being*. Advance online publication.

Bowker, R. M., Van Wulfen, K. K., Springer, S. E., Linder, K. E., & De Lahunta, A. (1995). Sensory nerve fibers and receptors in equine distal forelimbs and their potential roles in locomotion. *Equine Veterinary Journal*, *27*(S18), 141–146.

Bowker, R. M., Van Wulfen, K. K., Springer, S. E., Linder, K. E., & De Lahunta, A. (1993). Sensory receptors in the equine foot. *American Journal of Veterinary Research*, *54*(11), 1840–1844.

Bradshaw, R. A., & Dennis, E. A. (Eds.). (2009). *Handbook of Cell Signaling* (2nd ed.). Academic Press.

Breton, J., & Robertson, E. M. (2013). Memory processing: The critical role of neuronal replay during sleep. *Current Biology*, *23*(18), R836–R840.

Brubaker, L., & Udell, M. A. R. (2016). Cognition and learning in horses (Equus caballus): What we know and why we should ask more. *Behavioural Processes*, *126*, 121–131.

Buchheim, A., Heinrichs, M., George, C., Pokorny, D., Koops, E., Henningsen, P., & Gundel, H. (2009). Oxytocin enhances the experience of attachment security. *Psychoneuroendocrinology*, *34*(9), 1417–1422.

Budiansky, S. (2012). *The Nature of Horses: Exploring Equine Evolution, Intelligence, and Behavior*. Free Press.

Cabib, S., & Puglisi-Allegra, S. (2012). The mesoaccumbens dopamine in coping with stress. *Neuroscience & Biobehavioral Reviews*, *36*(1), 79–89.

Cavalleri, J. M., Klopfleisch, R., Jahnke, R., Gerhauser, I., & Distl, O. (2013). Morphometric magnetic resonance imaging and genetic testing in cerebellar abiotrophy in Arabian horses. *BMC Veterinary Research*, *9*, 105.

Ciftcioglu, U. M., Linden, J. F., & Kremkow, J. (2020). Visual information processing in the ventral division of the mouse lateral geniculate nucleus of the thalamus. *Journal of Neuroscience*, *40*(26), 5019–5032.

Clegg, H. A., Freire, R., & Nicol, C. J. (2008). The ethological and physiological characteristics of cribbing and weaving horses. *Applied Animal Behaviour Science*, *109*(1), 68–76.

Corbetta, M., & Shulman, G. L. (2002). Control of goal-directed and stimulus-driven attention in the brain. *Nature Reviews Neuroscience*, *3*(3), 201–215.

Crossley, M. (2019). Proactive and retroactive interference with associative memory consolidation. *Communications Biology*, *2*, 368.

Crowell-Davis, S. L. (1993). Social behavior of the horse and its consequences for domestic management. *Equine Veterinary Education*, *5*(3), 148–150.

Cybaluk, N. F., & Christison, G. I. (1989). Effects of diet and climate on growing horses. *Journal of Animal Science*, *67*(1), 48–59.

DesRoches, A. D., Richard-Yris, M. A., Lemasson, A., Henry, S., & Hausberger, M. (2008). Laterality and emotions: Visual laterality in the domestic horse (*Equus caballus*) differs with objects' emotional value. *Physiology & Behavior*, *94*(3), 487–490.

Dias, B. G., & Ressler, K. J. (2014). Parental olfactory experience influences behavior and neural structure in subsequent generations. *Nature Neuroscience*, *17*(1), 89–96.

Dinot, S. V., & Cohen, N. D. (2013). Epigenetic regulation of gene expression: Emerging applications for horses. *Journal of Equine Veterinary Science*, *33*(3), 193–202.

Draaisma, R. (2020). *Language Signs & Calming Signals of Horses*. CRC Press.

Eagleman, D. (2015). *The Brain: The Story of You*. Vintage Books.

Eichenlaub, J.-B., Hétru, S., Bertran, F., Rueda-Delgado, L. M., & King, J.-R. (2020). Replay of learned neural firing sequences during rest in human motor cortex. *Cell Reports*, *31*(5), 107789.

Emery, B. (2010). Regulation of oligodendrocyte differentiation and myelination. *Science*, *330*(6005), 779–782.

Farmer, K., Krüger, K., & Byrne, R. W. (2010). Visual laterality in the domestic horse (*Equus caballus*). *Animal Cognition*, *13*(2), 229–238.

Feinstein, J. S., Adolphs, R., Damasio, A., & Tranel, D. (2011). The human amygdala and the induction and experience of fear. *Current Biology*, *21*(1), 34–38.

Fiedler, D., Reiser, M., Weitlauf, C., & Ratté, S. (2021). Brain-derived neurotrophic factor/tropomyosin receptor kinase B signaling controls excitability and long-term depression in oval nucleus of the BNST. *Journal of Neuroscience, 41*(3), 435–445.

Flagel, S. B., Clark, J. J., Robinson, T. E., Mayo, L., Czuj, A., Willuhn, I., Akers, C. A., Clinton, S. M., Phillips, P. E. M., & Akil, H. (2011). A selective role for dopamine in reward learning. *Nature, 469*, 53–57.

Floyer-Lea, A., & Matthews, P. M. (2004). Changing brain networks for visuomotor control with increased movement automaticity. *Journal of Neurophysiology, 92*(4), 2405–2412.

Frank, D. W., Harper, D. N., & Phelps, E. A. (2014). Downregulation and upregulation: Slower modulation of the total number of receptors present in cells or tissues. *Neuroscience and Biobehavioral Reviews, 45*, 202–211.

Freymond, S. B., Briefer, E. F., Zollinger, A., Gindrat-von Allmen, Y., Bachmann, I., & Hillmann, E. (2015). The physiological consequences of crib-biting in horses in response to an ACTH challenge test. *Physiology & Behavior, 151*, 121–128.

Fuentemilla, L., Miró, J., Ripollés, P., Vilà-Balló, A., Juncadella, M., Castañer, S., ... Rodríguez-Fornells, A. (2013). Hippocampal-dependent strengthening of targeted memories via reactivation during sleep in humans. *Current Biology, 23*(18), 1769–1775.

Fureix, C., Jego, P., Henry, S., Lansade, L., & Hausberger, M. (2011). Co-occurrence of yawning and stereotypic behavior in horses (*Equus caballus*). *Zoology, 114*(3), 181–188.

Furr, M., & Reed, S. (2007). *Equine Neurology* (1st ed.). Wiley-Blackwell.

Fuster, J. M., & Alexander, G. E. (1971). Neuron activity related to short-term memory. *Science*, *173*(3997), 652–654.

Gallo, E. F., Meszaros, J., Sherman, J. D., Chohan, M. O., Teboul, E., Chuhma, N., ... Kellendonk, C. (2018). Accumbens dopamine D2 receptors increase motivation by decreasing inhibitory transmission to the ventral pallidum. *Nature Communications*, *9*, 1086.

Gleerup, K. B., Forkman, B., Lindegaard, C., & Andersen, P. H. (2015). An equine pain face. *Veterinary Anaesthesia and Analgesia*, *42*(1), 103–114.

Grahn, J. A., Parkinson, J. A., & Owen, A. M. (2009). The role of the basal ganglia in learning and memory: Neuropsychological studies. *Behavioural Brain Research*, *199*(1), 53–60.

Greening, L., McBride, S. D., & Tallo-Parra, O. (2021). The effect of altering routine husbandry factors on sleep duration and memory consolidation in the horse. *Applied Animal Behaviour Science*, *236*, 105242.

Hall, C., Huws, N., White, C., Taylor, E., Owen, H., & McGreevy, P. (2013). Assessment of ridden horse behavior. *Journal of Veterinary Behavior*, *8*(2), 62–73.

Heehler, T. (2025). *The Well-Spoken Thesaurus*. Source Books.

Hipp, J., Arabzadeh, E., & Diamond, M. E. (2006). Texture signals in whisker vibrations. *Journal of Neurophysiology*, *95*(3), 1792–1799.

Horvitz, J. C. (2009). Stimulus-response and response-outcome learning mechanisms in the striatum. *Behavioural Brain Research*, *199*(1), 129–140.

Houpt, K. A., Houpt, T. R., & Johnson, J. L. (2001). The effect of exercise deprivation on the behavior and physiology of straight stall-confined pregnant mares. *Animal Welfare, 10*(3), 257–267.

Iigaya, K., Ahmadian, Y., Sugrue, L. P., Corrado, G. S., Loewenstein, Y., & Newsome, W. T. (2018). Effect of serotonergic stimulation on learning rates for rewards apparent after long intertrial intervals. *Nature Communications, 9*, 2477.

Insel, T. R. (2010). The challenge of translation in social neuroscience: A review of oxytocin, vasopressin and affiliative behavior. *Neuron, 65*(6), 768–779.

Jackson, J. (2016). *Paddock Paradise: A Guide to Natural Horse Boarding*. James Jackson Publishing.

Jeffrey, D. (1996). *Equine Gnathology: Horse Dentistry, Balance Through Range of Motion*. World Wide Equine.

Johnson, P. J., Wiedmeyer, C. E., Messer, N. T., & Ganjam, V. K. (2012). Diabetes, insulin resistance and metabolic syndrome in horses. *Journal of Diabetes Science and Technology, 6*(3), 534–554.

Keeling, L., Jonare, L., & Lanneborn, L. (2009). Investigating horse-human interactions: The effect of a nervous human. *Veterinary Journal, 181*(1), 70–71.

Keleman, Z., Janczarek, I., Wilk, I., & Stachurska, A. (2021). Recumbency as an equine welfare indicator in geriatric horses and horses with chronic orthopaedic disease. *Animals, 11*(11), 3291.

Kiley-Worthington, M. (2009). Stereotypic behavior in stabled horses. *Equine Veterinary Science, 6*, 49–54.

Krakauer, J. W. (2008). Consolidation of motor memory. *Trends in Neurosciences, 31*(1), 58–65.

Kurlan, R., Shoulson, I., Rubin, A. J., & Lichter, D. (1982). Up- and down-regulation: Clinical significance of nervous system receptor–drug interactions. *Clinical Neuropharmacology, 5*(4), 345–350.

Lahunta, A., Glass, E., & Kent, M. (2014). *Veterinary Neuroanatomy and Clinical Neurology* (4th ed.). Saunders.

Lakhani, B., Borich, M. R., Jackson, J. N., Wadden, K. P., Peters, S., & Boyd, L. A. (2016). Motor skill acquisition promotes human brain myelin plasticity. *Neural Plasticity, 2016*, Article 7526135.

Lansade, L., Bouissou, M. F., & Erhard, H. W. (2005). Effects of neonatal handling on subsequent manageability, reactivity and learning ability of foals. *Applied Animal Behaviour Science, 92*(1–2), 143–158.

Leblanc, M. (2013). *The Mind of the Horse: An Introduction to Equine Cognition*. Harvard University Press.

Lewis, K. P., Mench, J. A., & Mason, G. J. (2022). Risk factors for stereotypic behavior in captive ungulates. *Proceedings of the Royal Society B: Biological Sciences, 289*(1974), 20212244.

Luke, K. L., Minero, M., Baragli, P., & McLean, A. (2022). New insights into ridden horse behavior, horse welfare and horse-related safety. *Applied Animal Behaviour Science, 246*, 105539.

Lupien, S. J., Maheu, F., Tu, M., Fiocco, A., & Schramek, T. E. (2007). The effects of stress and stress hormones on human cognition: Implications for the field of brain and cognition. *Brain and Cognition, 65*(3), 209–237.

Ma, S., & Morilak, D. A. (2005). Norepinephrine release in medial amygdala facilitates activation of the hypothalamic-pituitary-adrenal axis in response to acute immobilization stress. *Journal of Neuroendocrinology*, *17*(1), 22–28.

Maier, S. F., & Seligman, M. E. P. (1976). Learned helplessness: Theory and evidence. *Journal of Experimental Psychology: General*, *105*(1), 3–46.

Mal, M. E., Friend, T. H., Lay, D. C., Vogelsang, S. G., & Jenkins, O. C. (1991). Physiological responses of mares to short-term confinement and social isolation. *Journal of Equine Veterinary Science*, *11*(2), 96–102.

Mayhew, I. G. (2008). *Large Animal Neurology* (2nd ed.). Wiley Blackwell.

McBride, G. E., Christopherson, R. J., & Young, B. A. (1985). Metabolic rate and plasma thyroid hormone concentrations of mature horses in response to changes in ambient temperature. *Canadian Journal of Animal Science*, *65*(1), 187–194.

McEwen, B. S. (2015). Preserving neuroplasticity: Role of glucocorticoids and neurotrophins via phosphorylation. *Proceedings of the National Academy of Sciences*, *112*(51), 15544–15545.

McFarlane, D., Holbrook, T. C., & Thatcher, C. D. (1998). Hematologic and serum biochemical variables and plasma corticotropin concentration in healthy aged horses. *American Journal of Veterinary Research*, *59*(10), 1247–1251.

McGowan, C. M., & Hyytiainen, H. K. (2017). Muscular and neuromotor control and learning in the athletic horse. *Institute of Veterinary Science*.

McGreevy, P. (2004). *Equine Behavior: A Guide for Veterinarians and Equine Scientists.* Saunders.

McGreevy, P. D., Cripps, P. J., French, N. P., Green, L. E., & Nicol, C. J. (1995). Radiographic and endoscopic study of horses performing an oral-based stereotypy. *Equine Veterinary Journal, 27*(2), 92–95.

Mellor, D. J., & Reid, C. S. W. (1994). Concepts of animal well-being and predicting the impact of procedures on experimental animals. In R. Baker, G. Jenkins, & D. J. Mellor (Eds.), *Improving the Well-Being of Animals in the Research Environment* (pp. 3–18).

Mendelsohn, D., Riedel, W. J., & Sambeth, A. (2009). Effects of acute tryptophan depletion on memory, attention, and executive functions: A systematic review. *Neuroscience & Biobehavioral Reviews, 33*(6), 926–952.

Molyneux, G. S., Halleran, J., & Phillips, T. J. (1994). The structure, innervation and location of arteriovenous anastomoses in the equine foot. *Equine Veterinary Journal, 26*(4), 305–312.

Motta, S. C., Carobrez, A. P., & Canteras, N. S. (2017). The periaqueductal gray and primal emotional processing critical to influence complex defensive responses, fear learning and reward seeking. *Neuroscience & Biobehavioral Reviews, 76*(Pt B), 39–47.

Murphy, B. A. (2019). Circadian and circannual regulation in the horse: Internal timing in an elite athlete. *Journal of Equine Veterinary Science, 76,* 14–24.

Neimark, M. A., Andermann, M. L., Hopfield, J. J., & Moore, C. I. (2003). Vibrissa resonance as a transduction mechanism for tactile encoding. *Journal of Neuroscience, 23*(16), 6499–6509.

Nicol, C. (1999). Understanding equine stereotypies. *Equine Veterinary Journal, 31*(S28), 20–25.

O'Keefe, J., & Dostrovsky, J. (1971). The hippocampus as a spatial map. *Brain Research, 34*(1), 171–175.

Olds, J., & Milner, P. (1954). Positive reinforcement produced by electrical stimulation of septal area and other regions of rat brain. *Journal of Comparative and Physiological Psychology, 47*(6), 419–427.

Ousey, J. C., Rossdale, P. D., Palmer, L., Fowden, A. L., & Short, C. E. (1992). Thermoregulation and total body insulation in the neonatal foal. *Journal of Thermal Biology, 17*(1), 1–10.

Park, H. R., Park, M., Choi, J., Park, K. Y., Chung, H. Y., & Lee, J. (2010). A high-fat diet impairs neurogenesis: Involvement of lipid peroxidation and brain-derived neurotrophic factor (BDNF). *Neuroscience Letters, 482*(3), 235–239.

Peters, A. J., Chen, S. X., & Komiyama, T. (2017). Learning in the rodent motor cortex. *Annual Review of Neuroscience, 40,* 77–97.

Porges, S. W. (2011). *The Polyvagal Theory: Neurophysiological Foundations of Emotions, Attachment, Communication, and Self-Regulation.* W. W. Norton & Company.

Racklyeft, D. J., & Love, D. N. (1990). Influence of head posture on the respiratory tract of healthy horses. *Australian Veterinary Journal, 67*(11), 402–405.

Rajendra, A. M., Dennis, E. L., & Thompson, P. M. (2012). Amygdala volume changes with post-traumatic stress disorder in a large case-controlled veteran group. *Archives of General Psychiatry, 69*(11), 1169–1178.

Ramey, P. (2011). *Care and Rehabilitation of the Equine Foot*. Hoof Rehabilitation Publishing.

Rees, L. (2017). *Horses in Company*. J. A. Allen.

Riccarda, W., Hausberger, M., & Möstl, E. (2018). Parameters for the analysis of social bonds in horses. *Animals, 8*(11), 191.

Riedel, W. J., Klaassen, T., Deutz, N. E. P., van Someren, A., van Praag, H. M., & Blokland, A. (2002). Tryptophan, mood, and cognitive function. *Brain, Behavior, and Immunity, 16*(5), 581–589.

Rivera, E., Benjamin, S., Nielsen, B., Shelle, J., & Zanella, A. J. (2002). Behavioral and physiological responses of horses to initial training: The comparison between pastured versus stalled horses. *Applied Animal Behaviour Science, 78*(2), 235–252.

Rizzolatti, G., & Luppino, G. (2001). The cortical motor system. *Neuron, 31*(6), 889–901.

Rochais, C., Fureix, C., Lesimple, C., & Hausberger, M. (2016). Investigating attentional processes in depressive-like domestic horses (*Equus caballus*). *Behavioural Processes, 124*, 93–96.

Rogers, L. J. (2023). Knowledge of lateralized brain function can contribute to animal welfare. *Frontiers in Veterinary Science, 10*, 1140633.

Rotter, J. B. (1954). *Social Learning and Clinical Psychology*. Prentice-Hall.

Sapolsky, R. M. (2004). *Why Zebras Don't Get Ulcers* (Rev. ed.). St. Martin's Press.

Sara, S. J. (2009). The locus coeruleus and noradrenergic modulation of cognition. *Nature Reviews Neuroscience, 10*(3), 211–223.

Sarrafchi, A., & Blokhuis, H. J. (2013). Equine stereotypic behaviors: Causation, occurrence, and prevention. *Journal of Veterinary Behavior: Clinical Applications and Research, 8*(5), 386–394.

Saunders, B. T., & Robinson, T. E. (2012). The role of dopamine in the accumbens core and expression of Pavlovian-conditioned responses. *European Journal of Neuroscience, 36*(4), 2521–2532.

Schmidt, M. J., Kramer, E., Oevermann, A., & Kircher, P. R. (2019). Neuroanatomy of the equine brain as revealed by high field (3 Tesla) magnetic-resonance-imaging. *PLOS ONE, 14*(4), e0213814.

Shafir, T. (2016). Using movement to regulate emotion: Neurophysiological findings and their application in psychotherapy. *Frontiers in Psychology, 7*, 1451.

Shipp, S. (2017). The functional logic of corticostriatal connections. *Brain Structure and Function, 222*(2), 669–706.

Shreiner, A. B., Kao, J. Y., & Young, V. B. (2015). The gut microbiome in health and in disease. *Current Opinion in Gastroenterology, 31*(1), 69–75.

Siegel, D. J. (1999). *The Developing Mind: How Relationships and the Brain Interact to Shape Who We Are*. The Guilford Press.

Singer, A. C., & Frank, L. M. (2009). Rewarded outcomes enhance reactivation of experience in the hippocampus. *Neuron, 64*(6), 910–921.

Squire, L. R., Berg, D. E., Bloom, F. E., du Lac, S., Ghosh, A., & Spitzer, N. C. (2012). *Fundamental Neuroscience* (4th ed.). Academic Press.

Squire, L. R. (2015). Memory consolidation. *Cold Spring Harbor Perspectives in Biology, 7*(8), a021766.

Stanley, A. T., Ghosh, R., Jarvie, B. C., & McElligott, Z. A. (2023). Norepinephrine release in the cerebellum contributes to aversive learning. *Nature Communications, 14*, 4852.

Stoessl, A. J. (1994). Dopamine D1 receptor agonist-induced grooming is blocked by the opioid receptor antagonist naloxone. *European Journal of Pharmacology, 259*(3), 301–303.

Talukdar, A. H., Getty, R., & Ghoshal, N. G. (1972). Microscopic anatomy of the skin of the horse. *American Journal of Veterinary Research, 33*(12), 2365–2390.

Takeuchi, T., Duszkiewicz, A. J., & Morris, R. G. M. (2016). The locus coeruleus and dopaminergic consolidation of everyday memory. *Nature, 537*(7620), 357–362.

Todeschinia, A. S., Winkelmann-Duarte, E. C., Jacob, M. H. V., Aranda, B. C., Jacobs, S., Fernandes, M. C., & Sanvitto, G. L. (2009). Effects of neonatal handling on social memory, social interaction, and number of oxytocin and vasopressin neurons in rats. *Hormones and Behavior, 56*(1), 93–100.

Tononi, G., & Cirelli, C. (2006). Sleep function and synaptic homeostasis. *Sleep Medicine Reviews, 10*(1), 49–62.

Van de Kamp, N., van den Hoven, R., & Gmel, A. I. (2020). EEG-based assessment of stress in horses: A pilot study. *PeerJ, 8*, e8629.

Vatistas, N. J., Snyder, J. R., Carlson, G., Johnson, B., Arthur, R. M., Thurmond, M., Zhou, H., & Lloyd, K. L. (1999). Cross-sectional study of gastric ulcers of the squamous mucosa in thoroughbred racehorses. *Equine Veterinary Journal Supplement, 31*(29), 34–39.

Whitfield-Cargile, C. M., Cohen, N. D., Chamoun-Emanuelli, A. M., Brady, C. M., & Fragoso, J. (2021). Effects of phenylbutazone alone or in combination with a nutritional therapeutic on gastric ulcers, intestinal permeability, and fecal microbiota in horses. *Journal of Veterinary Internal Medicine, 35*(2), 1121–1130.

Wickens, C. L., Heleski, C. R., & McBride, S. D. (2010). Crib-biting behavior in horses: A review. *Applied Animal Behaviour Science, 128*(1–4), 1–9.

Wilkinson, M., & Brown, R. E. (2015). *An Introduction to Neuroendocrinology* (2nd ed.). Cambridge University Press.

Williams, J. L., Friend, T. H., Nevill, C. H., & Archer, G. (2003). Effects of imprint training procedure at birth on the reactions of foals at age six months. *Equine Veterinary Journal, 35*(2), 127–132.

Yang, Y., & Lisberger, S. G. (2014). Purkinje-cell plasticity and cerebellar motor learning are graded by complex-spike duration. *Nature, 510*(7506), 529–532.

Zaghloul, A. A., Khalil, M. R., Soliman, M. A., & Elbadawy, M. (2024). Comparative pharmacokinetics of phenylbutazone in healthy adult-young and geriatric horses. *American Journal of Veterinary Research, 85*(8), 1–8.

Zatorre, R. J., Fields, R. D., & Johansen-Berg, H. (2012). Plasticity in gray and white: Neuroimaging changes in brain structure during learning. *Nature Neuroscience, 15*(4), 528–536.

Zhang, X., Liu, Y., Li, J., Gao, C., Wang, Y., & Wang, J. (2025). Dopamine induces fear extinction by activating the reward-responding amygdala neurons. *Proceedings of the National Academy of Sciences, 122*(18), e2319173121.

Zhu, S., Jiang, Y., Xu, K., Wang, L., & Wang, W. (2020). The progress of gut microbiome research related to brain disorders. *Journal of Neuroinflammation, 17*, 25.

ABOUT THE AUTHOR

Dr. Stephen Peters, MS, Psy.D., ABN, is a neuroscientist and board-certified clinical neuropsychologist dedicated to applying neuroscience insights to horse training and care. He completed his practicum at Abbott Northwestern Hospital, an internship at Danbury Hospital, and a two-year postdoctoral fellowship at Hartford Hospital, in the departments of Neurorehabilitation, Neurology, and Neurosurgery. For over a decade, he served as Chief of Neuropsychological Services in a large Neurology practice, where he participated in clinical research trials using strict scientific protocols. Dr. Peters also founded and held the position of Clinical Director of The American Fork Hospital Memory Clinic and the Utah Valley Hospital Clinic for Brain Health.

Now retired from clinical practice, Dr. Peters combines decades of experience in brain research with his passion for horses. Through his *Horse Brain Science Clinics* offered worldwide, he shares his expertise through classroom sessions, equine brain dissections, and live demonstrations. Renowned for his ability to translate complex scientific concepts into practical, easy-to-understand information, he empowers horse enthusiasts and professionals alike, including those without a scientific background, to deepen their understanding of equine behavior, learning, and welfare through equine neuroscience.

A sought-after keynote speaker and presenter at scientific and medical conferences, Dr. Peters is co-author of *Evidence-Based Horsemanship* with Martin Black and author of *The Book of Neuropoetry*, a pioneering fusion of neuroscience and poetic expression.

Dr. Peters lives at River Rock Ranch in Mancos, Colorado, with his wife, Michelle, their Australian Shepherd, Kippi, and their seven horses—Comet, Bug, Jodi, Skadi, Takoda, Cassidy, and Ruby. To learn more about his work and Horse Brain Science Clinics, visit *Horsebrainscience.info*.

www.ingramcontent.com/pod-product-compliance
Lightning Source LLC
Chambersburg PA
CBHW022055160426
43198CB00008B/244